Fat and Happy?

Weight Loss Strategies for People Who Love to Eat

By

Dr. Doug Pray

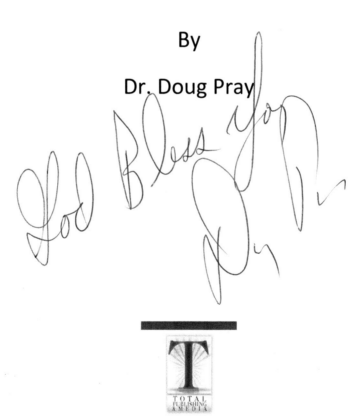

www.TotalPublishingAndMedia.com

ISBN: 978-1-936750-31-3

This book is dedicated to my mother, Nita Creekmore, who helped me from the start on my weight loss journey

And to my wife and partner, Jill, who continues to support and inspire me

Endorsement

After graduating high school I weighed over 300 pounds and addicted to junk food. I would have given anything to become thin and kick my food addiction, I just didn't know how and every time I tried I failed. I came across Dr. Pray's book *I Don't Go With Fat Boys*, this book was a game changer for me. I identified so much with Dr. Pray and his struggles with his own food addiction that I felt like I was reading a story about my life. It was time for a new beginning for me and I decided to try the cleanse program and follow the healthy lifestyle Dr. Pray wrote about. I ended up losing 11 pounds during my initial 7 day cleanse. After following the lifestyle that Dr. Pray recommends I have been able to keep losing weight and keep it off, after two years of regular cleanses, chiropractic adjustments and healthy lifestyle choices I now weigh 175 pounds. As a pleasant surprise to me, the lifestyle changes that I have made have also gotten me off of a nasal steroid that helped me breathe for nearly 15 years and now without any medication I can breathe better than ever! Thanks to Dr. Pray I am a much more confident person and I am a better husband, father and friend who truly enjoys life to its fullest.

Table of Contents

Introduction

Many of you who read my first book, "I Don't Go With Fat Boys -- Weight Loss for People Who Love to Eat", say how much you appreciate me sharing my story and what I have learned about the underlying causes of the unhealthy lifestyles that have created our overweight society. You say, after reading "I Don't Go With Fat Boys", you better understand the "why" of your roller coaster weight struggle. Now you would like some practical "how tos" for successfully achieving and maintaining your weight goals and gaining health for yourselves.

I very much want you to know that I have struggled with weight my entire life, and this book comes from my personal search for answers to my own weight and health issues. I am one of you. I know exactly the struggles you experience. I am not one of those people who have always done it right.

Our youngest daughter, Melissa actually says she needs to go for a run when she feels stressed. Where does that come from? When I feel stressed, I say, "I need to eat a pint of Chunky Monkey ice cream". Reality is, most foods available today are unhealthy choices, and those foods are my natural inclination.

I have developed ways to help myself make better choices, but I do slip at times, and I have to work out answers for when I fail to stay with my plan. I have examined the mind and behaviors of a food junkie like myself, and created strategies for me, and those like me, who find making healthy food choices difficult.

My purpose in sharing this book with you is to encourage you, and let you know you are not alone in this battle. There are many of us who are seeking to stay the course toward weight loss and improved health. When we get off track, we experience feelings of failure and hopelessness. We come to believe we will never succeed, but that is not *truth*!

This book does not offer a perfect plan. In fact, I don't believe there is such a thing as a perfect plan. *Truth* is, there are simple strategies that can help us stay our course, and answers for when we slip off-track that will help get us back up and moving forward again.

Blessings Always,
Dr. Doug Pray

Chapter 1

It's Easy?

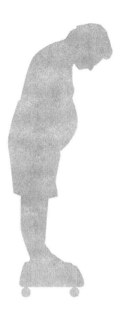

For most of us, the hardest part of any change in eating habits is sticking with our new plan when life gets hectic. A diet plan that supplies prepackaged meals seems like an easy solution, but is ineffectual at producing lasting change. If we don't learn to make satisfying meals from healthy foods, we won't be able to maintain our weight loss once our "diet" is over. This book is all about making the right decisions when faced with difficult circumstances, such as meals out with friends or preparing a meal at the end of a particularly busy day. And when we slip, and we all do, we must put it in perspective and take steps to get ourselves back on track.

We all face the difficulties of a fast-paced lifestyle. Recently, I found myself in one such circumstance. My wife, Jill and I have a good friend who is a massage therapist. Once a month, she gives Jill and me a massage and then stays for dinner, which I usually have waiting when their session is finished. As I was leaving the office on this particular day, I realized that we had nothing at home to cook. I had less than an hour to pick up groceries, get home and have dinner ready. Between traffic and the distance to my home, I knew that if I stopped at the grocery store I wouldn't have time to prepare anything before the ladies were ready to eat. So I ran into a convenience store. I know what you're thinking, "Really, Doug? You expect us to believe you found ingredients for a healthy dinner at a convenience store?" It is true most foods in convenience stores have little or no nutritional value. I'm certainly not suggesting you do your weekly shopping at the corner gas station. I tell you this to demonstrate that if you have a tight schedule and limited options you can still find a way to make a healthy meal that is delicious and filling.

While browsing the isles, I came across some cans of soup. I bought two cans of potato soup that had about 250 calories each. With the base for my evening meal secured, I raced home, emptied the soup into a pot and set it on the stove to heat. Now, I knew that canned soup was not going to give my wife and our friend the nutritional value, much less the taste they expected. I checked the freezer. I keep a variety of frozen vegetables in the freezer and in about five minutes I can add a very healthy component to a meal. I opened a bag of broccoli-carrot-cauliflower mix, and dropped the contents into the soup.

I let the soup simmer while I worked on what I think is an essential component to any meal, the presentation. Instead of grabbing mismatched bowls, I set the table with china and crystal glasses. I opened a bottle of red wine and set out the silverware and cloth napkins. Then, with the mood set, I checked on my soup. It was simmering and filling the kitchen with a delicious aroma. I remembered we had a few new potatoes in the pantry. I quickly washed the potatoes, sliced them, dropped them into a bowl of water, and popped it into the microwave. After a few minutes the potatoes were ready to add to my soup, which had started as a couple of cans from a convenience store and now was filling my home with the sensuous aroma of a delicious home cooked meal. I tasted the soup and realized it was a little bland, so I added some garlic salt and black pepper and let it continue to simmer while I cleaned up the kitchen.

In less than half an hour I had prepared dinner, set the table with a wonderful presentation, and cleaned up after myself. I wanted to finish off our meal with dessert. In the pantry, I found a can of sliced peaches and another of sliced pears. I opened both cans, rinsed off the syrup, and spooned the fruit into crystal bowls. I put the bowls of fruit into the refrigerator to chill, and checked on my soup. It was perfect. I spooned out generous helpings into our bowls. As the ladies entered, I poured them each a small glass of red wine and a glass of cold water. My wife and our friend were delighted with the soup. They complimented me on how delicious and hearty it was and how great everything looked. Both of them had second helpings and sipped their wine as I went to the kitchen to finish dessert. Taking the chilled fruit from the refrigerator, I lightly sprinkled it with sugar and cinnamon. Most people don't know that a heaping teaspoon of sugar has less than 25 calories. Cinnamon is a great source of iron, calcium, fiber and manganese. It has been shown to lower LDL cholesterol and fight E. coli bacteria. Some studies have shown that the smell of cinnamon boosts cognitive function and memory. I like it because it tastes so good, and just a light dusting on fruit makes a delicious and simple dessert. The ladies were thrilled that I had taken the time to prepare such a wonderful meal and raved about my dessert.

In less than an hour I had stopped at a convenience store, made my way home, prepared a wonderful meal, and best of all, even though the ladies had two helpings of the soup, they still consumed less than 500 calories, even with dessert.

You may be thinking that you can't make meals on the fly, or that you just don't know how to make eating healthy work. I'm here to tell you that with a few simple tricks and some staples to keep in your house, you can become a wizard of healthy eating and cooking, without spending hours in the kitchen or a fortune on groceries. Eating right is not about being perfect, it's about doing the best you can and not giving up. Every day is an opportunity for you to live healthier, happier and stronger lives. Each day that we eat right we extend our lives just a little, and we enjoy the blessings of life a little more.

In this book, I'm going to show you how to do it. It only takes a little time and a little know how. Before you know it, you'll be preparing the best meals of your life in less time than it takes to watch your favorite television show.

Cajun Chili

1 medium onion – chopped
1 red pepper – chopped
1 large tomato – chopped
1 can (15oz.) kidney beans
1 Tbs. garlic powder
1 Tbs. chili powder
1 tsp. paprika
1 tsp. thyme
1 tsp. oregano
1 tsp. cumin
¼ tsp. cayenne pepper

Using a little juice from the canned tomatoes, sauté onions and peppers 5 minutes, stirring frequently. Mix tomatoes, beans and cooked ingredients in a pot. Mix in spices and simmer over low heat 30 minutes. Serve hot with Kale Chips.

Kale Chips

1 bunch kale

Wash kale and cut off stems. Dry completely, and cut leaves into thirds. Lay out leaves on cookie sheet and bake 10 minutes at 375 degrees. Leaves will be light and crispy.

This recipe is great and the best choice to serve with homemade chili. But, to prepare this same type of chili meal in our real life experience, rushing home with kids from ball practice, getting homework started and throwing in a load of laundry, what I have been known to do is reach into the cabinet and prepare, in less than 5 minutes (time me, I dare you!), a "whatever is in the cabinet homemade chili" consisting of one can of black beans (rinsed), one can of pinto beans (rinsed), one can of petite diced tomatoes (with juice), a hand full of corn flakes (or rice flakes) crushed by hand and thrown in, and half a package of chili seasoning mix. The kale chips are wonderful, but remember we are keeping this meal to less than 5 minutes preparation time. Instead of kale chips you can substitute a small handful of BAKED potato chips. This will feed a family of four one hearty serving each. If you are big eaters make it double and you are still less than 500 calories per meal. Oh, are you wondering why the corn flakes? They give the chili a light corn flavor and make it appear to have meat. So, you have cooked a great vegetarian chili, and though not perfect, it is much healthier (and cheaper) than running by the fast food joint and grabbing meals for everyone.

Baked Lemon Pepper Fish with Pea Puree

1 pound fresh fish
2 Tbs. lemon juice
1 Tbs. black pepper
1 tsp. garlic powder
1 bag frozen green peas
1 medium onion – diced
1 cup chicken or vegetable broth
4 Tbs. sunflower seeds
¼ tsp. salt

Preheat oven to 400 degrees. Rub fish with lemon juice and sprinkle with garlic powder and black pepper. Place in baking dish and bake 20 minutes. Meanwhile, sauté the onion with a spoonful of broth 5 minutes, stirring frequently. Add the remaining broth, peas, salt and sunflower seeds and simmer an additional 4 minutes. Place pea mixture into blender and puree until smooth. Serve fish with pea puree on side.

At first glance this recipe may sound like "YUCK!" But, it tastes great, is fairly quick to prepare, very low in calories, and packed with nutrition, including essential fatty acids. A winner all around!

Sautéed Chicken and Vegetables

1 large bag mixed vegetables (or 2 bags of steam-in-microwave vegetables)
1 pound free range chicken – diced.
¼ cup water
1 tsp. garlic salt
1 tsp. black pepper

Steam vegetables. Heat water in skillet and add chicken. Sauté chicken 8 minutes, stirring frequently. Spoon vegetables onto plate and top with chicken. Sprinkle chicken and vegetables with garlic salt and pepper.

Mushroom Topping

1 cup dried porcini mushrooms - sliced
1 cup Crimini mushrooms – sliced
1 cup white onion – diced
2 cloves garlic – minced
2 Tbs. chicken or vegetable broth

Heat broth in sauté pan until steam is visible. Cook onions 5 minutes, stirring frequently, then add mushrooms, and garlic. Continue cooking another 3 minutes. Serve over Sautéed Chicken and Vegetables (or over any lean meat or potato dish)

This is an absolutely wonderful healthy and hearty meal. But, in the spirit of time saving, yet still healthy (remember we talk a lot about choosing well and compromise), you could open a can of mushroom soup, heat and pour over your chicken and veggies. Not as savory and decadent but still one cup of mushroom soup is only 160 calories, so your meal remains under 500 calories. Yum, making healthy choices and cooking quick meals can be fun and scrumptious.

Bonus 5 minute meals: Don't have time to prepare a meal? Grab ingredients on your way home or fix them from whatever is in the pantry.

Dr. Doug's Chili on the Fly

1 can black beans rinsed
1 can red beans rinsed
1 can pinto beans rinsed
1 can diced tomatoes (seasoned or plain) with juice
1 pkg of chili seasoning

Pour rinsed beans and tomatoes with juice into a cooking pot. Add 1 pkg of chili seasoning. Keep a variety of seasoning mix packages on hand for quick meal preparation. Cook till boiling, then simmer. This makes a great vegetarian chili, if you like meat add ½ pound lean ground beef or turkey browned. When you brown meat separate your servings into smaller portions and put in freezer bags to be used when in a hurry. A very inexpensive meat substitute is a ½ cup of crushed corn flakes. The cooked flakes look like ground meat and give the chili a light corn flavor.

Dr. Doug's Stew on the Fly

1 can low sodium beef broth
1 can diced or chopped tomatoes
1 can black beans
1 can mixed vegetables
1 small potato diced
1 pkg stew seasoning mix

Bring beef broth to a boil in stew pot. Add diced or chopped tomatoes, rinsed black beans, rinsed mixed vegetables, diced potato and ½ pkg stew seasoning mix. Let simmer. If you like meat in your stew, add whatever leftover piece of meat (beef, chicken, turkey, etc.) you have in your refrigerator, chop and add to stew.

Chapter 2

Eat Right

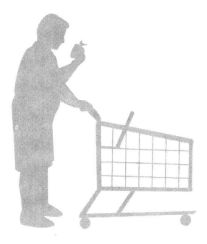

I was 12 years old when I discovered that I had a weight problem. Over the next 45 years I have tried all the diets and fads, lost weight and gained it back, and finally, through research and study developed a plan for living healthy and losing weight that really works. I call it Choose Right, Eat Right, Move Right. This plan is laid out in detail in my book *I Don't Go With Fat Boys – Weight Loss for People Who Love to Eat.* I want to take some time in this chapter to review the plan, although this book is more about putting the plan into practical use rather than educating you on the plan itself.

I'm a Chiropractic Physician, and many of my patients come to me in hopes that I can help them lose weight. In the last two decades I've coached hundreds of people to success in losing weight. In fact, most of my patients lose weight and keep it off. But not because Choose Right, Eat Right, Move Right (CEM) is a quick fix or even a diet in the normal sense of the word. CEM isn't something you do for twelve weeks and then go back to eating all the things that got you overweight in the first place. That yo-yo method of weight loss never works. CEM is all about making better choices. And while the idea of making lifestyle changes may be scary or daunting, A healthy lifestyle is attainable, in fact this book will show you how. And the great thing about CEM is that you don't have to starve yourself thin, you don't have to count calories, or order special meals, or spend a fortune in diet club memberships. It's simply about making better choices in what you eat. When you're eating the right foods you can eat as much as you want. So let's see what CEM is all about.

Most people don't realize that our bodies are amazing machines, created to keep us healthy. Unfortunately, we live in a toxic world where much of the things around us can make us sick. Our bodies do a great job of filtering out the toxic junk that we're exposed to everyday, but because of the abundance of toxic food and chemicals in our world, our bodies become overwhelmed. Imagine if everyone in your city wanted to see the band that was playing at the local high school. As more and more people arrived to see the show, the school would quickly run out of room. They might have to offer an overflow room to accommodate all those extra people. Our bodies are similar to that. Our liver is an incredible organ that filters the toxic junk from the good stuff in what we eat and drink. But due to the high content of toxins in our foods, our livers are overwhelmed and need to store the surplus toxins somewhere. The body's two favorite places to store excess toxins are in fat cells and neural tissue (that's your brain!). It doesn't take a degree in biochemistry to see why Americans are so unhealthy.

Let's take a look at what I mean when I say that much of the foods we eat are filled with toxins. Take bread for example. Most people eat sliced sandwich bread, sometimes several times a week. But have you ever taken a look at the ingredients in your average loaf of bread? There's a long list of words that leave no doubt that they aren't natural ingredients, things like sodium stearoyl lactylate, monocalcium phosphate, dough conditioners and ammonium sulfate. How did the world bake bread without those chemicals for thousands of years? And take a look at our all-American food for the ill, chicken noodle soup. With ingredients like ferrous sulfate, monosodium glutamate, and sodium phosphates, there may be more side effects from chicken soup than from some prescription drugs. Toxins are everywhere, in our food, in our water, in the air we breathe, in the lotions and cosmetics we use. They're in our toothpaste, our deodorant, the sunscreen we use to protect us from harmful solar radiation, the paint on our walls, the stain protectors on our carpets and furniture, and of course all the cleaners we use in our homes.

If that sounds a bit scary, stick with me. I don't want to sound like an alarmist because we do have to live in this world. I want you to understand how bad the situation is, but in reality we do have to compromise. The best way to help your body deal with toxic overload is to eat nutrient-rich whole foods whenever possible. Eating nutrient-dense whole foods, and only those foods is of course the best choice. However, we have to live in our real lives every day and must learn to make the best choices possible in busy and sometimes difficult to manage situations.

Eating healthy whole foods is plain common sense. Whole foods are simply foods that haven't been messed with, there's nothing added, no chemicals or flavor enhancers or preservatives. What about fortified foods you ask? Fortified foods sound good, I mean aren't they adding needed vitamins and minerals to our food? Actually, in most cases, fortified foods have been stripped of all their natural nutrients. The producers add or fortify the foods with chemically produced vitamins and minerals to make their products legally classifiable as nutrition sources again. Imagine trading peanuts for Styrofoam packing that's been fortified, which would you choose? The reason most of us eat so much is because our bodies are starving for basic nutrients. We're eating enough calories but not getting the nutrient benefits that our bodies require.

Whole foods allow us to take in what our bodies need, resulting in better health, while keeping our appetites satisfied longer. The **Nutrient Density Scale** (following and Appendix I), is a scale developed by Dr. Joel Fuhrman, a medical doctor and whole food expert practicing in New Jersey. This list rates foods according to the ratio of nutrients to calories. In creating his Nutrient Density Scale, Dr. Fuhrman considers a thousand calories of a particular food, and then calculates all the nutritional components of that food. He assesses the content of protein, fats, carbohydrates, water, vitamins, minerals and phytonutrients (plant nutrients). The greater the content of each and every nutritional component, the higher the food is ranked on his scale. Foods high on this scale are foods packed with the most nutrition per calorie.

A sample of Dr. Fuhrman's Nutrient Density Scale:

Kale	1000	Cucumbers	50
Collards	1000	Soybeans	48
Bok Choy	824	Sunflower Seeds	45
Spinach	739	Brown Rice	41
Cabbage	481	Salmon	39
Red Pepper	420	Shrimp	38
Romaine Lettuce	389	Skim Milk	36
Broccoli	342	White Potatoes	31
Cauliflower	295	Grapes	31
Green Peppers	258	Walnuts	29
Artichoke	244	Bananas	30
Carrots	240	Chicken Breast	27
Asparagus	234	Eggs	27
Strawberries	212	Low Fat Yogurt	26
Tomatoes	164	Corn	25
Plums	157	Almonds	25

Blueberries	130	Whole Wheat Bread	25
Iceberg Lettuce	110	Feta Cheese	21
Orange	109	Whole Milk	20
Cantaloupe	100	Ground Beef	20
Flax Seeds	44	White Pasta	18
Tofu	86	White Bread	18
Sweet Potatoes	83	Peanut Butter	18
Apples	76	Apple Juice	16
Peaches	73	Swiss Cheese	15
Kidney Beans	71	Potato Chips	11
Green Peas	70	American Cheese	10
Lentils	68	Vanilla Ice Cream	9
Pineapple	64	French Fries	7
Avocado	64	Olive Oil	2
Oatmeal	53	Cola	1
Mangoes	51		

For a complete list go to drjoelfuhrman.com

Simply put, the higher the nutrient density, the better the food is for you. It's like getting more for your money. Eating 200 calories of cantaloupe during the ballgame will give you almost ten times the nutrition as eating 200 calories of potato chips. And every bite is making you healthier rather than compromising your health, making you gain weight, and addicting you to unhealthy, processed foods.

The biggest challenge for most of us isn't knowing what we should eat, it's overcoming our addiction to refined foods – refined sugars and refined fats. Most of us don't choose our food options based on what is good for us, but rather on what tickles our taste buds. We've cultivated cravings for foods loaded with fat and processed sugars. Even though the abuse of food is just as deadly and addictive as alcohol or drugs, it's often overlooked or seen as acceptable in our society. What makes food addiction even more difficult to overcome is the fact that we must eat. You can't just avoid restaurants and only associate with thin people. With food, we have to train ourselves to choose healthy. Unfortunately our busy schedules and social customs make it even harder to eat right. We're surrounded by quick and easy solutions to our hunger: fast foods, prepackaged or frozen dinners, and highly processed foods that have a longer shelf life than fresh, whole foods. Even when it comes to our budgets, the wrong food choices are easy to rationalize than more expensive healthy foods. It's no wonder we're addicted to hamburgers that are loaded with fat, french fries cooked in refined oils, candy and ice cream desserts loaded with refined flour and sugar. Even diet drinks with chemical sweeteners are addictive. I knew a man named Todd who battled his weight and got hooked on diet sodas. He told me he craved them even when he wasn't thirsty. This phenomenon is linked to the chemical sweetener in the soda which triggers an insulin reaction in the body and actually makes a person crave carbohydrates. To satisfy this craving people eat or drink more. The artificial sweetener actually is contributing to weight gain!

So how do we break our addictions and poor diet choices and get rid of the toxins stored in our body tissues? That is the first step in my CEM plan. Eating right begins with a 7-day detoxification, or a cleansing of our filtering organs. Basically, detoxification is a way to flush out surplus toxins and give your body a chance to break the addiction to refined foods. The good news is that most people lose weight while they detox. Most women lose between 8-10 pounds and men usually lose between 10-12 pounds. At the end of a 7-day detoxification you should have more energy, be thinking more clearly and best of all, your pants will fit better.

What does a 7-day detoxification cleanse look like? Well, I'm not talking colon cleanse, so don't fear. I am referring to cleansing your filtering organs; your liver and kidneys, and ridding your body of the toxins stored in your fat and brain tissues. When toxins are released, your brain works better and your thought processes are clearer. Your body functions better when your brain can relay messages more efficiently. When toxins are released from fat cells, your body can more efficiently break the cells down and burn them for fuel. One of the duties of fat cells is to bind up toxins and buffer the body from their harmful effects. When the toxins are released and flushed from the body, the fat does not have to hang around to do that buffering job any longer so it is more easily broken down and metabolized. Your liver and kidneys are designed to trap toxins as they filter your blood as they filter the blood. If these filtering organs are clogged, they cannot work efficiently. When these organs are flushed, your body begins to work better and your overall health begins to improve.

I helped develop a 3-component detoxification and cleanse system that targets the release of toxins in a gentle yet highly effective process. The 7-day system includes a nutritional cleansing product, Ultra Cleanse, which is an all-natural formula that helps release toxins stored in your fat cells, your brain and neural tissue, and in your liver and kidneys. Each day you enjoy three meal replacements. These Energizer Protein shakes keep your body fueled and give you energy. Metaboost capsules continue the cleansing process and help boost your metabolism to burn off excess fat. To review the medical research related to the ingredients or to order a 7-Day Detoxification and Cleanse kit, visit http://www.novolife.net

Once you've jump started with the detoxification, you'll find your body actually craving healthy foods. No, really, you will crave good healthy foods. I know you don't believe it but over and over, patients tell me they are amazed that they actually crave foods like broccoli or spinach when they had never before wanted to eat them. Once you have cleansed, it's all about making healthy choices in what you eat. That sounds easy, but we know that in the real world the temptation to make unhealthy choices is great. We are bombarded with unhealthy, addictive, refined foods every single day. We will do the very best we can but we will slip. We are human and we do want to enjoy some of the "sinful" foods at times. Remember, I love to eat, and I love to eat the poor choices too. When you do slip up, and you will, you don't have to feel that you have failed. There is an easy answer and I will share that with you further in this book. In the meantime, I encourage you to try the following healthy recipes after you complete your 7-Day Cleanse.

Easy Vegetable Soup

4 cups water
1 large bag frozen vegetables
1 large tomato - chopped
½ tsp salt
½ tsp onion powder
½ tsp garlic powder
pepper to taste

Bring 4 cups water to boil in large pot. Add frozen vegetables and allow water to return to boil. Add tomato and spices and mix well. Reduce heat and simmer until soup is desired consistency. Serve hot.

Spicy Shrimp

½ pound medium shrimp – peeled and deveined
2 Tbs. lemon juice
3 Tbs. chicken or vegetable broth
2 cloves garlic - minced
1/8 tsp. red pepper flakes
¼ cup orange juice
1 Tbs. ginger - minced
Salt
Pepper

Rub shrimp with lemon juice then sprinkle with salt and pepper. Heat broth over medium-low heat. When broth begins to steam, add shrimp, garlic, red pepper flakes, orange juice and ginger. Sauté about 3 minutes, stirring frequently.

3-Minute Scallops

½ pound bay or sea scallops
2 cloves garlic – minced
1 Tbs. chicken or vegetable broth
½ cup green onions – finely chopped
1/8 tsp. sea salt

Heat broth in skillet. Add scallops, garlic, and green onions. Sauté 2 minutes then turn scallops. Sauté another minute then remove scallops. Drizzle with broth, garlic and onions. Serve hot.

Fig and Spinach Salad

½ medium onion – thinly sliced
2 Tbs. white wine or apple cider vinegar
1 cup hot water
8 oz. baby spinach
2 Tbs. balsamic vinegar
½ tsp. honey
8 dried figs – diced
2 Tbs. walnuts - chopped
Salt
Pepper

Marinate onions in hot water and wine or vinegar 5 minutes. For dressing, mix balsamic vinegar, honey, salt and pepper. Toss onions, spinach, walnuts and figs, drizzle with dressing and serve.

Sautéed Cauliflower

1 pound cauliflower
5 Tbs. chicken or vegetable broth
2 Tbs. cilantro – chopped
1 tsp. turmeric
Salt

Heat broth until it begins to steam. Add cauliflower and turmeric. Cover and simmer 5 minutes. Sprinkle with cilantro and salt. Serve hot.

Chapter 3

Food Addiction

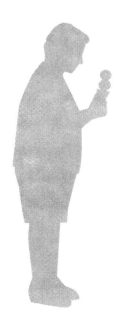

R emember the Lays potato chips commercial where the announcer says, "Bet you can't eat just one?" Guess what, you CAN'T eat just one. And the food companies are betting on that fact because they know the power of food addiction and they know the combination to create addictive foods. The combination of salt, fat and sugar (carbohydrate) is so strongly addictive to your mid brain that it can have a hold on you stronger than crack or cocaine. Oh, you say, it can't be that bad. Well, the effects may not be so rapidly evident as those seriously addictive substances but let me assure you, refined foods are just as addictive and deadly, though the effects may take years to manifest. And the ability to break free of the addiction is just as difficult. Food addiction is one of the deadliest problems to plague us in the modern world. We have children as young as two years old being diagnosed with obesity and health related problems such as diabetes, high blood pressure, liver and kidney failure. This is a serious problem and the sad thing is that it is preventable if we would only stop feeding our children refined addictive foods.

As I was developing the CEM program, I realized that the biggest obstacle most people face (including myself) is food addiction. One afternoon, I set out to test myself. Could I eat just one potato chip? I thought I was mentally tough; I thought I had strong will power. So I ate a chip, then a couple more, and I thought to myself, *Okay, that's enough.* I went into the living room and flipped on the television. Pretty soon I was thinking about that bag of potato chips. I really wanted to eat some more. You know how it is: the salty flavor as you pop it into your mouth, the crisp snap as you bite down, the way they just seem to magically flow from the bag to your tummy. I thought, *Well, just a few more won't hurt me.* So I got up, went back to the kitchen and got myself a small handful. I enjoyed those chips and then patted myself on the back for stopping after eating a reasonable amount. It wasn't long before I was thinking of the chips again. Oh, man, it was like they were calling my name. I wasn't hungry. I didn't need to eat, but I wanted those chips. Soon I was in the kitchen for just a few chips more. And then, after yet another trip I decided it would be much easier to take the bag back to the sofa with me. And you know the rest of the story: I ate the whole bag. It wasn't because I didn't know better, I absolutely did. It wasn't because I was hungry. I knew that I wasn't. Think about it. Why are potato chips so highly addictive? I've never heard of anyone being addicted to eating carrots or snap peas. Once you are full you stop eating. Still, most of the foods we buy precooked and packaged, are loaded with salt, fats and refined sugar. That deadly addictive combination causes us to gain weight and have weight related health issues.

Some of you may balk at this, you may be thinking I've gone too far, but take a moment and really consider the power food has over us. How many times have you sat at home after a sensible dinner and just craved something salty or something sweet? It isn't a matter of being hungry; in fact if we learn to listen to our body's needs we will find that junk food isn't something our body wants. Have you ever heard of people who are starving to death wanting dessert? No, they long for nutritious food. And if you've ever done a 7-day detox, or tried fasting, you know that foods high in salt, fat and refined sugar don't sound good. How ironic it is, that when we're starving we know what we need to eat, and when we're well fed we choose to eat foods with hardly any nutritional value.

After my experiment, I felt all the usual feelings with which poor food choices leave us. First of all there was the sick feeling of having overeaten. My stomach was bloated, I felt a little nauseous, I couldn't get comfortable on the couch, and it was as if someone had given me a sleeping pill. Sounds a lot like getting drunk doesn't it? And there were also the mental after-effects. I felt guilty for having failed my own test. I couldn't believe with all I know about food and nutrition that I had just eaten a whole bag of potato chips. I felt helpless to ever change my own bad habits. I felt like a hypocrite for teaching others to eat correctly and then giving in to my own food addictions. I was angry that I even had the chips in my house to tempt me (I promptly blamed that on my wife, looking for blame is a great escape from responsibility). The craziest part was that after all the guilt and feeling physically sick, my mind was already thinking of the next binge, perhaps a bag of cookies or a carton of ice cream.

That's the way addictions work. People don't do drugs and smoke cigarettes because they don't know any better. Alcoholics don't want to start their day with booze, but they can't help themselves. Even while they partake of their vice they are planning and dreaming about a little more or the next time. Food can become distorted in our minds and have very real physical reactions with our bodies beyond just added weight. That is why a diet that just removes certain kinds of foods never really works. We have to break our addiction to unhealthy foods if we want to live a healthy life.

Most of us can't afford to check ourselves into a center to detox from food and learn good eating habits. That's okay, because we don't need an escape or have someone else force us to eat healthy foods. What we really need is a good plan that is realistic and attainable. And of course we need a way to deal with the emotional and physical obstacles that trip us up. None of us are perfect, in fact I encourage my patients not to try to be perfect (I'm certainly not); trying to be perfect only sets us up for failure. Instead we need to try to live by the 90% rule. Eating right 90% of the time is attainable, we can all do that with a little effort and the occasional misstep won't send us careening off the safe and narrow path. Let me give you another example of how easy it is for me to foul up, and what I do when that happens.

Spending time with my grandchildren is one of my greatest pleasures. Not long ago, my wife, Jill, and I had our grandson, Gavin, overnight. Let's face it, getting a four-year-old to eat healthy isn't all that easy, and as you can probably guess, having a sugary breakfast cereal in our home isn't such a good idea for me. Normally, I start my day with a protein shake for breakfast. I knew my grandson would have none of that, so we took him to a local restaurant with a large breakfast menu where we could all find something we wanted to eat. It would not surprise you to know that most items on the menu were not healthy choices, but there were a few good options. I ordered a couple of poached eggs (the healthy alternative to fried eggs) and a fruit bowl. I was feeling pretty good about myself when my wife ordered biscuits with sausage gravy. Of course, I knew that she knew her breakfast choice was not healthy, so being the magnanimous man I am, I kept my mouth shut and simply gave her a "knowing look". She promptly informed me she would eat what she wanted. Properly chastised, I ordered my grandson the Mickey Mouse pancakes.

Our food soon arrived, and I quickly finished my poached eggs and fruit bowl. I was completely satisfied. My grandson was also finished, and he had left about half of his pancake. It was covered with maple syrup and butter, and I believe that Mickey was calling my name. I decided to have just one bite. After all, I had been so good in choosing the healthy breakfast. But, as you've probably guessed by now, stopping with just one bite was never my strong suit. Soon, I had eaten the rest of the pancake. And my wife, who had divided her large plate of biscuits and sausage gravy and eaten half, was giving me the other half of her breakfast. I wasn't even hungry but I couldn't stop eating. Sure, I had all the usual rationalizations in my back pocket, like the fact that I was already paying for the food, so I might as well eat it, there was no sense in letting it go to waste (even though it was now going to my waist). Besides, this was a special occasion. But of course I knew I was blowing it. That's not unusual for me. I love food.

This is the point where most diets fail, even my own, because of the addictive nature of food. Once we've put some distance between us and the addictive foods (salt, fat and refined sugar), a little taste reawakens all those cravings we've suppressed. It's much like the alcoholics my church works with. It can be tempting for them to have a beer when they're out with friends, especially when they've gone for awhile without any alcohol. But one beer inevitably leads to another and another, and before they know it, they wake up somewhere after being on a three-day binge and they have to suffer through the symptoms of detox all over again. We already know our best weapon for defeating food addictions is the 7-day cleanse, but one bad choice doesn't call for that kind of drastic action. The complete 7-day program is recommended three or four times a year to keep our body free from the harmful effects of toxins but not necessary to get us back on track after a poor-choice day or weekend. So, I developed a mini-cleanse system for quickly getting back on track. If I mess up for a day, I go on a 1-day mini-cleanse. If I go away for a weekend and eat things I shouldn't, I go on a 2-day mini-cleanse. This is simply doing the day-one process or the days one and two of the full-cleanse system. A mini-cleanse puts my addictive cravings back in check and I can continue on with healthy eating as I had before I messed up. It is the first time I have ever had a plan for getting back on track when I foul up, and it removes much of the guilt and self-loathing associated with eating binges. Some of my nutritional colleagues disagree with me. They say I am giving people permission to cheat. Well, let me tell you, everyone will cheat at some point, we can't be perfect at this, and we need an answer for when we do. I developed an answer because I needed one the same as everyone else. A mini-cleanse is especially useful in dropping that extra pound we pick up from a night out with friends and perhaps more importantly it gives us power over our cravings. Overeating can sneak up on us while we're not watching and steal away everything we've worked so hard to achieve. The mini-cleanse helps us stick to our guns when the cravings come to call.

After getting a speeding ticket several years ago I made up my mind not to bend the rules anymore. I decided that as much as it was in my power I would drive the speed limit at all times. Too often in my past I would glance down at the speedometer and realize that I was going five or even ten miles per hour over the speed limit, especially when I was on the highway. Isn't it funny how that speed never seems too fast from our perspective behind the wheel, just like a little bit more food, a few more bites, or one more slice never seems like too much food when we're eating? Before I made my decision not to speed I would often just continue on. Five miles over the limit would soon become ten, and then fifteen or even twenty. Now things are different; if I glance down and see that my speed exceeds the limit I immediately slow down and I almost always set my cruise control to ensure that I don't go too fast. In the same way, if you have a contingency plan and strategies for helping yourself stay on track in place before you slip up, you are much more likely to get your eating back under control.

A preventive plan for not messing up is perfect. Try not to tempt yourself with poor food choices. I think of one Sunday when the family was all home and enjoying the afternoon. The grandkids were playing and we were watching the Food Channel on television. A show celebrating the best hotdogs in America was playing. At first we laughed at all the great combinations but, before it was over we had made a list of all of our favorite ingredients and were headed to the store for supplies for our own hotdog cookout. My daughter, Auburn, was telling me just the other day that she can't even watch that channel because it makes her want to eat all of the things she tries so hard to avoid. So, even though creating habits that help us avoid being tempted is the best plan. We know, as my family did, we give in to the temptation at times. We have to have a plan for those occasions.

I recommend following the 1-day mini-cleanse with a day of greens, but if you're like me, salads can get old fast. I like to have a hearty, meal, something hot and tasty. A loaded baked potato makes a good meal that doesn't take long to prepare and will really fill you up. You can bake them in the microwave in about the time it takes to cook a frozen dinner. Just puncture the potato skin with a fork all around, wrap the potato in wet paper towels and then with microwaveable plastic wrap. Cook the potato on high about eight to ten minutes. People ask me about potatoes, because they are lower on the nutrient density list. It is not that they are poor nutrition, but rather, they lack a variety of nutrients. They are very low in calories and by adding green veggies to them you are boosting the nutrients of the overall meal. So go with potatoes when you wish, add vegetables to increase the nutritional value, just don't fry them!

In the meantime, prepare some broccoli to give your meal additional flavor, fiber and a nutritional punch. Steam frozen or fresh broccoli while the potato cooks, or even steam frozen broccoli in the microwave. Place broccoli in a microwaveable bowl, add a small amount of water, cover, and cook about five minutes. The potato with broccoli is very satisfying and contains less than two hundred calories. At that rate, you can have two potatoes if you want. And for extra flavor, add salsa or hot sauce. You can use bottled, as long as it isn't loaded with sugar, or try making the following Salsa recipe.

Salsa

2 large, red tomatoes
1 clove garlic
1 Anaheim green chili
¼ cup green onions
3 jalapenos
½ cup fresh cilantro
1 lime or ¼ cup lime juice
1 tsp extra virgin olive oil
Salt
Pepper

Grill (or roast in oven) the tomatoes, green chili and jalapenos. After cooling, peel the tomatoes. Devein and seed the green chili and jalapenos (this makes the salsa milder). In a food processor, chop the tomatoes, garlic, green chili, green onions, jalapenos and olive oil. Brush down the insides of the processor with a rubber spatula or spoon. Then set the food processor to puree and add the fresh cilantro and lime juice. Pour salsa into a bowl and add salt and pepper. Let the salsa rest for about an hour to allow the flavor to properly meld before serving.

Fajita Lettuce Wraps

2 boneless, skinless chicken breasts
1 medium onion - diced
1 medium bell pepper - diced
1 cup mushrooms – sliced
1 Tbs. chicken or vegetable broth
1 head butter lettuce
1 Tbs. fajita seasonings

Heat grill to medium. Sprinkle chicken breasts liberally with fajita seasonings. Grill 5 minutes on each side. Set aside and allow to cool. Heat sauté pan and broth to medium high heat, add bell pepper and cook, stirring frequently about 2 minutes. Add onions and cook 3 minutes. Add mushrooms and cook 2 minutes until all vegetables are soft. Dice chicken and mix with vegetables. Remove the outer leaves of the butter lettuce and then slice the entire head in half. Use individual leaves like tortillas, fill with chicken and vegetables and enjoy.

Ultimate Fruit Salad

2 cups of your favorite fruits – cut into small pieces
2 cups of your favorite dried fruit
2 cups of your favorite nuts or seeds

Mix fresh fruit, dried fruit and nuts together. Serve as a meal or in small portions as snacks.

Peanut Shrimp Salad

½ pound fresh shrimp – peeled and deveined
1 cup peanuts – coarsely chopped
1 head romaine lettuce – outer leaves removed
2 Tbs. lemon juice
2 Tbs. chicken or vegetable broth
½ tsp. garlic powder
2 Tbs. water
½ tsp. Italian herbs

Mix lemon juice and garlic salt together. Toss raw shrimp in mixture, then sauté in skillet with broth about 3 minutes. Cut off the bottoms of the romaine leaves and discard. Chop romaine and top with shrimp and peanuts. Mix water and Italian herbs. Drizzle over salad and serve.

Fruit Cocktail

4 large strawberries – washed and sliced
2 cups orange juice
1 banana – peeled
1 small can crushed pineapple

Mix all ingredients in a food processor and blend to desired consistency, serve chilled.

Chapter 4

Eating Right On Special Occasions

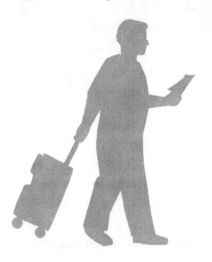

A s I write this, the holiday season is upon us. It's that mad and wonderful time of the year between Thanksgiving and Christmas. If ever there was a time to give up on a diet it's now. Face it, we've just feasted on all the Thanksgiving goodies, pies and candied foods. Then, right around the corner is Christmas and we're either eating as we enjoy the holiday, or eating just to get through the holiday; one sure thing is, we're eating. Most of us eat until we're stuffed and then graze on leftovers all week. Holiday parties are nonstop, and there's no such thing as a holiday health-food party. By definition, a party is where you leave your discipline and inhibitions at the door and do what feels good. Fatty, salty, sugary foods taste delicious and can knock us right back to square one in our effort to eat healthy.

So, how do we handle special occasions, nights out with friends, vacations or holidays? What should we do when we're only offered the very foods we're doing our best to avoid? The fact is, most of us can't resist, so let's just stop trying. Notice, I didn't stay that we should stop watching what we eat altogether. Let me give you a personal example.

A few months ago, Jill, and I went to Chicago for a weight loss conference with some of our very good friends. At the end of one very busy day, the question came up about where we should go for dinner. Now, I'm from Tulsa, Oklahoma, and we have some really good restaurants. But let's face it, Chicago is famous for great restaurants, especially pizza, the kind with thick crust, tons of cheese and heavenly sauce. So when someone suggested Gino's East Pizza (a place everyone visiting Chicago must eat), we all agreed. When we arrived at the restaurant, I knew I was in big trouble. Jill ordered a salad and one slice of pizza, for a total of about a thousand calories. That's right, I said ONE THOUSAND calories! I couldn't hold myself back. I ate three slices. Not only did I make the wrong eating choice, I overate to boot.

So, of course the next day I felt bloated and a bit ashamed, but when my friends suggested we go back to the same restaurant to try a different kind of pizza, I didn't even hesitate. By the time we left Chicago, I had gained a couple of pounds. Sound familiar? Sure, we've all done it and sometimes once we start we can't stop. How could something that tastes so great be so wrong? Actually, it has nutrition, it tastes wonderful, and in very limited quantities, it isn't all that terrible. The problem for most of us is, we don't have these foods only occasionally. We rationalize and find excuses, but the truth is, we're food junkies and we fall off the wagon. I'm a big proponent of the idea that food doesn't make us happy, but having fun and enjoying friends often involves food, and we shouldn't have to hide or exclude ourselves from the pleasures of life in order to have a healthy lifestyle. We just need to stop the yo-yo cycle of diets, start making healthy choices when we can, and have a plan in place for when we need a boost back on the wagon.

Later, we'll talk more about socializing with friends and food, but right now, let's get back to the holiday season, when we experience several days of overeating and poor food choices. If your mom is like mine, you know you will enjoy incredible traditional family foods and desserts for Thanksgiving and Christmas. In the past, I always stressed over how I would handle the holidays and eating. Now, I don't get panicky about what is served on those occasions. I eat and enjoy myself, because I know I have a plan in place to get myself back on track.

During my research, I came to understand that getting off-track by accident or knowing full well that I was going to mess up resulted in the same conclusion. I needed a solution to the problem of getting off-track. So, I developed a plan of action to take, (remember the mini-cleanse)? Let's start with the plan and then we'll talk about the mental attitude that makes the plan possible.

When I overate in Chicago, I came home two pounds heavier. No problem, I went on a 2-day mini-cleanse, followed by a day of green foods (if it's green eat it!). On the fourth day, I was THREE pounds lighter. I had lost the two I gained plus one! And, the cleanse helped rid my body of the "junk" I had ingested. Wow, now I'm ahead of the game. I enjoyed Gino's Pizza, I enjoyed time with my friends, and I ended up a pound down for the week. Finally, a solution for when I mess up. The mini-cleanse is my safety net for handling the occasional poor choices I make. Whenever I really fall off, as I occasionally do, I have an answer for that too. Let me tell you about a specific time I really messed up and I actually planned to mess up!

Our oldest son, Adam, and his family live in Egypt. So naturally, we planned a trip to visit. We knew we would be gone for about two weeks, and we would not be able to make great food choices much of the time we were gone. Traveling, airports, sightseeing and such, we were always in a place that did not offer a healthy variety of food choices. And, being in a country foreign from our own, we wanted to try all of the local dishes and desserts. We ate to our hearts' content, knowing full well, when we got back home we would have to address the results of all our gluttony. Upon our return, I was up seven pounds. Yikes! The next day I went on a full 7-Day Novolife Cleanse. That week reset my metabolism and relieved my addiction to refined and processed foods once again. In addition, I lost the pounds I had gained.

Wow, I had never before been able to live my life enjoying the special moments and events without worrying about breaking my healthy-eating habit. I can now stay motivated to choose healthy most of the time because I know I will not have to deprive myself when those special occasions occur, and when they do occur, I can get right back on track without losing my momentum.

Two important daily supplements that help me maintain my optimal weight and nutritional health are MetaBoost capsules and Energizer Protein

Meal replacement. The MetaBoost product assists in improving the body's fat burning ability and provides gently acting cleansing nutrients to prevent toxins from attaching to fat cells making them resistant to the metabolic process. I also replace one meal a day with the Energizer Protein Meal replacement. It helps reduce my overall daily calorie consumption. I am not a morning person, yet skipping breakfast is not a good idea, so typically, that is the easiest meal for me to replace. That way I don't need to plan ahead for a healthy breakfast. Some people tell me that lunch is their favorite meal to replace with the protein shake. They have a busy schedule and are not always in a place to choose a healthy lunch. The protein meal replacement solves their lunchtime dilemma. Still, others choose to replace their evening meal because, during the work week they get home late in the evening and don't have time to prepare dinner. The protein shake is the perfect answer. It provides all of the protein, carbohydrates, fats, fiber, vitamins, water and micro-nutrients necessary for a healthy meal.

However, it's important to understand how the Novolife system of products works so you don't fall into harmful thinking. The 7-Day Cleanse and the Mini-Cleanse solution isn't a fix all so you can binge whenever you want. That kind of thinking can lead to very harmful eating disorders that are no different than bulimia or anorexia. Our goal is to have a healthy lifestyle and binge eating is never healthy. You shouldn't go to holiday parties or special occasions intent on eating as much junk food as you can. You need to learn to enjoy food properly, and that means valuing how it feels to be *satisfied* rather than *stuffed*. The 7-Day Cleanse is not a fix-all for extended periods of overeating. In fact, the 7-Day Cleanse works best when used three to four times per year whether we are overeating or not. While you enjoy those times of allowing yourself to eat foods that are less healthy, it is important to make sure you are also including healthy choices. Knowing you will not always be forced to deprive yourself helps keep your mental attitude positive for making good food choices most of the time. The Novolife system of products is designed to help you enjoy a healthy lifestyle that is attainable and sustainable.

Peasant Soup

8 cups chicken broth
4 russet potatoes
2 cloves garlic
Kale, stemmed and chopped
1 carrot
1 large white onion
1 tsp olive oil
1 tsp salt
Pepper to taste

In a large pot heat the chicken broth. Wash and slice the potatoes leaving the skins on. Peel the carrot and then sliver, using peeler. Add potatoes and carrots to broth and cook 10 minutes, stirring occasionally. In a skillet, heat olive oil over medium heat and add onion (chopped) and garlic (minced). Cook about 5 minutes, stirring often. Add contents of the skillet to the soup and cook an additional 10 minutes. Remove the soup from heat and add salt and pepper. Ladle into bowls and add steamed chopped kale just before serving.

Why kale? Not only does it add an intriguing flavor, kale is known to be one of the most nutrient dense foods. And remember, nutrient dense foods are not just about lower calories and weight loss. Nutrient dense foods are the source of health and your body's ability to fight against disease.

Grilled Chicken with Squash and Zucchini

4 boneless, skinless, free-range chicken breasts
1 medium yellow squash – sliced
1 medium zucchini – sliced
½ cup green onion – chopped
1 tsp. chicken of vegetable broth
½ tsp garlic powder
1 pinch salt
Pepper to taste

Season chicken with salt and pepper. Grill over medium heat 10 minutes, turning once. Heat broth in skillet then add squash, zucchini and onions. Sauté, stirring frequently, for 6-8 minutes, then sprinkle with garlic powder. Serve with cooked chicken breasts.

Sweet Corn Salsa

2 large poblano peppers
2 cans whole kernel corn
1 cup white onion – diced
2 Tbs. lime juice

Preheat oven to 350 degrees. Roast peppers on a cookie sheet 10 minutes. Heat corn (with juice) in the microwave 3 minutes. When peppers are roasted, cut off stems and remove seeds, then chop peppers and mix with corn and onions. Toss with lime juice and chill half an hour. Serve cold.

Tomato Hash

2 large tomatoes – diced
1 cup red pepper – minced
1 cup green onions – finely chopped
1 cup whole kernel corn
1 cup black beans – drained and rinsed
1 cup cilantro - chopped
1 Tbs. chili powder
1 Tbs. cumin
1 tsp. salt

Over medium heat, scramble all ingredients together and cook 5 minutes. Serve hot.

Baked Sesame Crab Cakes

½ pound fresh crab meat
1 free-range egg
½ cup sesame seeds
½ cup peanuts
2 cloves garlic – chopped
¼ cup chicken or vegetable broth

Preheat oven to 350 degrees. Place all ingredients in food processor and blend. Form small patties and arrange in baking dish. Place in oven and cook 30 minutes.

Chapter 5

Eating Out

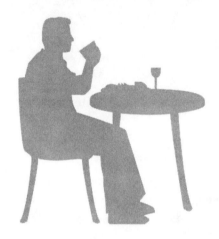

We all love to go out for a nice dinner. Unfortunately, for those of us who struggle with our weight, eating out can be a major stumbling block. It is difficult to be given a large portion of food and not eat everything set before us. Our culture has embraced mealtimes as social events. Fad diets make us feel fearful of going out with friends, and straining our relationships. Sometimes, we isolate ourselves to avoid temptation, only to end up "feeding" our need for companionship at home. I want to help you deal with the temptations of overeating and poor food choices so you can enjoy nights out with friends. I want people to see your healthy lifestyle and be motivated to make changes in their own lives. I want you to feel comfortable going out, knowing you are in control, and even when you slip, you have the tools and knowledge to pick yourself up and continue living a healthy life.

My friend Toby has a weakness for Mexican food. Most Mexican food restaurants offer free tortilla chips and salsa as an appetizer. While overeating fried chips is not a good idea, some people can enjoy a small helping, eat a small portion of their meal, and leave the restaurant full with a nice bit of leftovers for lunch the next day. But most people can't stop at a few chips, and the reason they can't stop, is the addictive nature of that deadly combo of salt, fat and sugar (the carbohydrate). Toby doesn't care for salsa. Instead, he loves to dip his chips into the cheese dip. Yum, but they're even more toxic when you add dairy to the deadly combo. He usually eats so many chips drenched in the rich cheese sauce that by the time his meal arrives he is completely full. Unfortunately, like many of us, he will often eat his entire dinner despite the fact that he is no longer hungry. No wonder he says he often feels sick after eating out, his stomach bloated and his body exhausted. All his energy is used up digesting the food with which he stuffed himself.

Sound familiar? It isn't uncommon to see people overeating in restaurants. Some people feel that not eating as much as they can is wasting money, even though they could actually save money if they take home half their food to be eaten as another meal. Others get carried away with socializing and overeat or over-consume alcohol as the evening progresses. Whatever the reason, eating out doesn't have to be a diet killer. I am as susceptible to making bad food choices and over-eating as the next person, but I refuse to hide from the problem. I believe if we face the issue head on, we can find ways to help ourselves avoid the pitfalls and still have a great time with family and friends.

The first lesson we need to remember is to never go out hungry. If you tend to overeat every time you eat out, then you need to keep your appetite light. Often, people who are looking forward to a night out with friends at their favorite restaurant, skip meals and put off their hunger, so by the time they reach the restaurant they're starving. Their ravenous hunger, combined with their love of the food, leads to disaster. Soon they've gorged themselves on pre-meal foods like chips and salsa, or buttery dinner rolls, and what most of us don't realize is that by filling ourselves up on these foods which are often high in salt, fat and refined sugar, we are actually activating the addictions that lead us to overeat. When we eat too much of the pre-meal foods, we are anesthetizing our taste buds, so the food doesn't taste as good, but our addictions drive us to eat anyway.

Can you remember when you were young and played outside in the hot summer afternoons? Oftentimes you would play until you were so thirsty you felt like you could drink a gallon of water. The thought of syrupy soda was repugnant. Do you remember how good water tasted on those days? It took on a sweet taste because it was exactly what our bodies needed. I can remember going to a week-long summer camp where the water had a distinct sulfur flavor. Sulfur water does NOT taste good. At first we would drink just enough to get by, but after an afternoon playing ball, even that tainted water tasted good. Our palate can be influenced by thirst and hunger. Have you ever stood in the kitchen, surrounded by food, feeling like you wanted to eat but nothing sounded good? That's because when we're full, food loses it's savor. But our addictions drive us to continue eating, searching for flavor satisfaction.

When we put off our hunger because we know we're going to dinner at our favorite restaurant, the normally bland fillers taste delicious. It's no different than water when you are extremely thirsty. So you end up eating the bland, pre-meal fillers until you can no longer enjoy the richness of the food you came to eat. It's like trying to pick up delicate flowers with thick winter gloves on your hand. It's impossible because the thick padding keeps you from feeling the stem with your fingers and forces you to squeeze so hard to get a grip that you end up crushing the beautiful flower. Overeating is the same, it keeps your palate from tasting the flavors and forces you to eat too much trying to satisfy your craving for the taste.

Instead of starving yourself in anticipation of a great meal, try eating a small snack before you go out. That way you don't hinder your appetite, but you don't set yourself up for failure before you even leave for dinner. An apple is an excellent choice for a pre-meal snack. Apples are both juicy and fibrous, which means they do a good job of suppressing the appetite without filling you up, and they cleanse the palate so that you can really enjoy all the tastes of your special meal. The fiber in apples also helps prepare your digestive track for richer foods. If you find yourself especially hungry right before a meal (or if the food preparation takes longer than you expect) drinking water is an excellent way to keep your hunger in check without filling you up.

Another reason people make bad eating choices when they go out is lack of attention paid to the food itself. Oftentimes when we eat out it is a social event and people are so busy talking, laughing and catching up they don't pay any attention to the food. Ever find yourself eating just because the food is in front of you? How many times have you heard someone say, take this away from me or I'll just keep eating it? We often feel that on nights out that we need to eat and drink the entire time, but that just isn't the case. If we can learn to enjoy the food, stop eating when we're full, and have the excess removed from the table in front of us, we'll end up much healthier. A simple glass of water can occupy our fidgeting hands just as well as a fork or spoon.

For those of you who feel leaving a restaurant without dessert makes the meal unfinished, try ordering dessert first. Even if you only have a bite before your meal, you'll find that you won't be as tempted to overeat just to work dessert into your dinner. And lets face it, ordering dessert first can only make you a more interesting person, and who wouldn't love to be more interesting?

For many of us, the amount of food we eat isn't as hard to control as what we eat. Just like our dessert lovers, most of the food we crave is anything but healthy. Eating at restaurants can be a minefield. Fortunately, many restaurants are adding healthy choices to their menus in hopes of catering to people who care about their diets. I highly recommend frequenting these establishments and letting management know why you chose their restaurant over the competition. It will encourage the restaurant owners to offer even more healthy options. Here are a few rules to remember when you eat out to help you avoid the kinds of food that will knock you backwards in your efforts to live a healthier lifestyle.

First, be choosey in where you eat. Just because you are going out with friends doesn't mean you have to eat at the same old greasy spoon. Look for restaurants that will give you good eating choices, it will make your job easier than trying to be happy with the one dish that isn't deep fried and loaded with calories, your usual place offers. I know that no one likes change, but variety is the spice of life so try a new place and I'll bet you'll have just as much fun without losing what you've worked for all week.

Second, small changes can make a huge difference in the amount of salt, fat and refined sugar you consume when you are eating out. We probably all know someone who carries their own salad dressing around. You may feel that pulling out a big bottle of fat free salad dressing just isn't you, and that's okay. Most bottled fat free dressings are loaded with chemicals and preservatives that wreak havoc on your body anyway. It's much easier to simply ask for a few slices of lemon, lime or other citrus fruit that most restaurants keep on hand. Squeeze the fruit juice onto your salad for a refreshing and bright taste that will keep you away from high fat oils and high calorie, creamy salad dressings.

Choosing grilled foods and light colored meat over dark or red meats. Do your best to order healthy sides, such as grilled vegetables over mashed potatoes or french fries, and tomato-based sauces instead of cheese-based sauces. Water can be flavored with the same fruit juice you squeezed over your salad, has no calories, and won't fill your stomach up with the carbonation in sodas and beer. When it comes to wine, have a glass of red over white. While white wine may seem to be lighter and therefore healthier, red wine in moderation has a health benefit such as antioxidants and resveratrol, an anti-inflammatory substance, which is good for your heart. Many restaurants have fresh fruit for dessert, which is a much better choice than cakes or pastries.

Also, keep in mind that we are striving to make good food choices as much as possible, not perfection. If you make a poor choice or eat too much, like I have done countless times, have your plan in place to stop the addictive food cravings and balance out your weight gain. Our goal is learning to eat healthy, not just continual dieting. Following are a few easy snacks to help curb your cravings before you go out and help you avoid poor food choices.

Apples – I keep mentioning apples and your first response may be *how boring*. Do I really expect you to be satisfied with an apple to snack on before going out for dinner? Well, did you know there are over 7500 varieties of apples worldwide? Try a variety you've never tasted. Mix things up and keep several varieties on hand. Apples may sound simple, but there's a lot more to this all-American fruit than meets the eye.

Nuts or Trail Mix – Small portions are great at curbing cravings and are loaded with healthy vitamins and minerals. Plus you have the added benefit of a hearty crunch, which can make a small amount of nuts or trail mix very satisfying. Because nuts take longer to digest, they are great at keeping you feeling full longer. Just be careful not to eat too much, as most nuts are high in calories.

Trail Mix Recipe

1 cup slivered almonds – lowers cholesterol, promotes weight loss and good for your complexion
1 cup chopped pecans – lowers cholesterol and inhibits cancer
1 cup raisins – improves eyesight, digestive health and increases energy
1 cup dried pineapple – boosts immune system and aides digestive health
1 cup dark chocolate chips – good for the heart, low in calories and tastes great

Mix all ingredients together in a large bowl until evenly distributed. Store in small (snack size) zip top plastic bags.

Dried Peas – are becoming more and more popular for their satisfying crunch and amazing health benefits. Dried peas are great for lowering cholesterol, regulating your blood sugar and are packed with antioxidants. You can find them with a wide variety of seasoning, just be sure to look for options that avoid sugar and excessive salt.

Chapter 6

Choosing Right

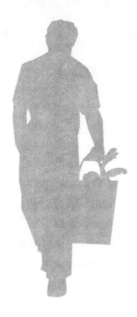

Life is all about making choices. We choose everyday, from the time we wake up, until we go to sleep at night. Most of us take our power of choice for granted. We don't often face choices that have a huge impact on our life. Usually, we face small, seemingly unimportant decisions, like what to wear, or which route to take to work. We don't think about small choices adding up like pennies, but over time they do. When we make poor choices about our health and what we eat, the consequences may seem small but over time they exact a heavy toll.

At a weight loss seminar I taught, I asked the group, "how many of you like being fat?" No one raised a hand; they were all there because they wanted to lose weight. When I told them they were choosing to be fat, there was an up-roar. They said things like, "they didn't want to be fat, they couldn't help themselves, it wasn't their fault". But as we began to examine what they ate on a regular basis it became clear that they were "choosing" to be fat. No one likes to admit it, but we make choices every day that affect our weight, even choosing how we think about food, about ourselves, and about our health. If we think we have no choice, we are trapped. If we think we can't change, we won't. But if we take responsibility for our actions, for our choices, then we can change, we can lose weight, and we can be healthy.

Imagine for a moment that you are a fish in a pond. You like the pond, there's plenty of food and space to swim. The pond is a calm place where you feel safe and have other fish friends. There are a lot of things within the pond that you have control of, like what you eat or where you swim. There are other things that you have no control over, like when someone stands on the shore and throws rocks into the pond. If you spend all your time worrying about the person throwing rocks you'll find yourself discouraged. You can't control that person, or even the other fish in the pond. But you do have total control of you. You have control of your choices. You control what you think about, what you do and how you do it.

I know that there are a lot of overweight people who feel that they can't control their eating. They feel helpless and out of control, like a runaway train that's off the rails. They blame their environment, or their health issues, their relationships or genetics for their unhealthy lifestyles. And, while some factors in our lives that affect our health may be beyond our control, there are always positive choices we can make. Let's take a look at some the choices over which we do have control.

Let's start with some obvious choices, like what kind of food you keep in your house. When you get hungry after a long day, and you open a pantry or refrigerator that is full of junk food, do you think it's reasonable to think you'll make a good choice? I know that many of you have spouses and children who insist on having highly fattening, refined foods on hand (do you really want them eating those foods either? well that is another issue). That may or may not be in your control, but even if it isn't, it is in your control to make a space that is just for your healthy, whole foods. You can choose to designate a cabinet or shelf in your refrigerator or pantry that is just for you. We'll talk later about healthy staples that you should keep on hand so that you can create quick and easy healthy meals. But right now, I just want you to ask yourself, if you never buy good foods, what choices are you making available for yourself?

How about your lunch on busy days? Do you find yourself struggling over fast food options? It's no wonder that we struggle with healthy eating when most fast food restaurants offer little or no good-food choices. We can't control what restaurants offer on their menus, but we can control what we eat for lunch. A little preparation time is all it takes to bring a healthy lunch with you whether you are at work, mother's day out, or even on vacation. It's your choice, no one is making you eat unhealthy foods, but let me fill you in on a little secret. If you find a way to bring healthy foods with you, you can eat as much and as often as you want, without all the debilitating side effects of unhealthy food. You'll feel energized and healthy while those around you are bloated, tired and unable to concentrate. And even more importantly, you'll be full!

Now, there are choices which probably way a little heavier on you, but they're still your choices to make. I know a guy who regularly spends five or six nights a week out with friends. I support any of you who enjoy a rich social life and I want to help you do what you love in a healthy way, but let's face it, few foods most restaurants offer are healthy choices. My friend may try his best to eat healthy, but a person who is eating out that often is going to find making the right choice very difficult.

Alcohol is also a difficult choice when it comes to maintaining a healthy lifestyle. We have a high-consumption culture and for many people, drinking is as much a part of a night out with friends as the socialization itself. Oftentimes, you may consume one drink after another while enjoying friends and not even realize the volume you are consuming. You probably didn't know that alcohol has 7 calories per gram (protein = 4 calories per gram; carbohydrates = 4 calories per gram; fat = 9 calories per gram). A typical cocktail has 200 calories, a glass of wine is 100 calories and a drink like a Long Island Tea can have up to 900 calories! Drinking a few drinks over the evening can easily add 1200 calories to you daily intake. Volunteer to be the designated driver more often and you'll be healthier and a hero to your friends.

Another complicated choice is finding healthy, whole foods at prices that fit your budget. If you're concerned about the price of food, I have two very encouraging bits of information for you. First, the thought that eating healthy has to cost you more money is a myth. Of course, you can choose to buy all your food from the trendy, organic only, health food store, but being wise about what you buy at mainstream grocery store will get you the same results and not bust your budget. With the rise in popularity of whole foods many grocery stores and super markets are carrying healthy food choices, you just have to look a little harder to find them. Also, local farmer's markets and co-ops often have very reasonably priced alternatives to the refined foods sold in bulk by the big chain stores. Additionally, when you buy healthy whole foods only, leaving the packaged and boxed foods out of your grocery cart, you actually spend less on your grocery budget.

Here is another bit of encouragement. Did you know that stress is one of the most common overeating triggers? By being budget smart (buying only the healthy whole foods and no packaged foods) and keeping your finances in order, you are lowering your stress level and the chances of financial hardship leading you to cope with food. You don't have to go broke to be healthy, but you do have to choose to buy the right foods.

Let's look at another area where our choices make a big impact on our health, and that is what we choose to think about. There are literally hundreds of books, videos, seminars and programs to help us keep a positive attitude, and that's because it's been proven that our thoughts control our life. The Bible says that as a man thinks in his heart, so *is* he (Proverbs 23:7a, italics added). So, what are you *choosing* to think about? Do you tell yourself you can never change? Do you say that you can't help yourself? When you give in to self-defeating feelings and thoughts, you are choosing to stay fat. Mental resolution is extremely important when it comes to making good choices about what you eat. If you are choosing to have a negative attitude while trying to make healthy choices you are just setting yourself up for failure. The way you choose to view yourself is the foundation for every action you take. It's important that you see yourself as a person with the power to choose.

Remember our comparison to the fish in the pond? If the fish tells himself that he'll never be happy because of the person throwing stones into the water, then even when there are no rocks being thrown that fish will squander its time in fear and trepidation. The fish will say, "I could go out and enjoy the pond, but sure as shooting, as soon as I do, that giant will start throwing rocks in the pond again". Do you see how our choices about who we are and what we can do affect us? Don't defeat yourself before you even get started. Choose to see that you have the power to choose.

In the movie "The Shawshank Redemption" Tim Robbins' character talks about music and how it reminds him that there is more to life than the walls of their prison. He had just spent several weeks in solitary confinement for playing an operatic aria, and the other characters asked him how he handled being alone all that time. Tim Robbins said that he wasn't alone, he had Mozart and the other classical composers to keep him company. He was trying to make the point that how you view your circumstances, especially the things that you can't control, is perhaps more important than the sum of your actions. In the movie, Tim Robbins' character has no control over what he does, or what he eats or where he goes. But he argues that his choice about what he thinks and believes is fully his to control. It's the same with us as we deal with the difficult circumstances of our health and face the confines of our poor choices and bad habits, but even then we can maintain our freedom by choosing to stay positive.

I've met a lot of people who tell me they don't like the taste of healthy food. The truth is they've befuddled their taste buds with high fat, high salt foods. They're like an addict who needs more and more drugs to get the same high. These people need more and more overwhelming flavor to get the tastes they want. They've allowed food addictions to rob them of the discernment that God has blessed us all with. It's why the French use sorbet between courses of their rich foods to cleanse the palate, so that they can taste the different flavors being presented. We have a daughter, Christin, who is a professional photographer. She takes a lot of pictures in black and white. I've learned by looking at the pictures with less color to notice the subtle shades and variations to the pictures she takes that would be lost in the myriad of colors of a high resolution, color photograph. Food is the same as color to our palate. When we eat whole foods, which are delicious and full of flavor (although admittedly less than highly refined foods), we begin to regain the power of taste.

For most of us, it begins at childhood. Children are understandably loath to eat vegetables because they often have flavors that are slightly bitter or earthy. Kids just want to eat foods that taste sweet. If we grow up shocking our palates, it won't be any wonder why we can't enjoy healthy foods as adults. Children who grow up never or rarely eating refined foods actually love vegetables.

Not enjoying the taste of healthy, whole foods is a choice. If you choose to eat candy bars and chocolate cakes, fruit will often seem repugnant, sour or tasteless. If you choose to overwhelm your palate with foods that are high in salt and refined fats, then vegetables will seem bitter and unappetizing. But if you break your addiction to refined food (which is a great benefit of the 7-Day Cleanse), you will notice flavors you never tasted before. Just as sweet and salty tastes complement one another, so do bitter and savory, earthy and tangy, acidic and gamey. It all comes down to how you choose to think about your food.

Do you want to be fat? No, none of us want to be fat, feel bad, get sick and hate the way we look. But wanting to make a change, and making the choice to change, is totally different. Remember, all those little choices we make everyday add up to who we are. If you're really ready to change, you have to choose not to be fat, and that choice affects what you do every day. Take some time to really think about the choices you make. And, never forget that you are not alone. You, alone, have had trouble for too long. Utilize the power that was born in you, "as a man thinks so *is* he". You and the power of God in you, have the control over your choices, not your friends or family, not your circumstances or even your limitations. You can make the choice today to be healthy and eat foods that are rich, satisfying and good for you. Here are some recipes to try when you're ready to make the choice to change!

Poached Eggs Over Spinach (or Kale)

2 free-range eggs
1 pound spinach (or kale)
1 tsp. vinegar
1 Tbs. lemon juice
½ tsp. garlic salt
½ tsp. pepper

Bring a large pot of water to a rapid boil. Submerge spinach for 1 minute exactly, and then drain water (if using kale see below). Mix lemon juice, garlic salt and pepper and toss over hot spinach. In a separate pan bring 1 quart of water and 1 tsp. vinegar to a simmer, reduce heat to keep water temperature constant. Crack eggs directly into the water and allow them to cook 5 minutes. Place eggs on top of warm greens and serve.

If using kale use steaming basket and steam chopped kale leaves (remove stems) 5 minutes.

Italian Frittata

3 free range eggs - beaten
1 medium onion, minced
1 medium tomato, seeded and diced
1 cup of thinly sliced mushrooms
2 cloves of garlic, pressed
2 Tbs. chicken or vegetable broth
3 Tbs. chopped fresh basil
Salt and pepper to taste

Using 1 tablespoon of broth, sauté onions 3 minutes. Add garlic and mushrooms and continue cooking 2 minutes. Add the remaining broth, tomato, salt and pepper and cook 1 minute. Turn heat to low, add eggs and basil, mix until all ingredients are evenly distributed. Cover and cook 5 minutes. Slice into wedges and serve.

Black Bean Chili

1 can (15oz.) black beans – drained and rinsed
1 med. onion
1 large tomato – diced
2 cloves garlic – diced
½ cup bell pepper - diced
2 Tbs. chili powder
1 bunch cilantro – chopped

Heat onions and garlic in pot 2 minutes, stirring frequently. Add beans, tomato, bell pepper and chili powder. Bring to a simmer then cover, reduce heat and cook 20 minutes, stirring occasionally.

Serve in bowls with chopped cilantro sprinkled on top.

Seared Tuna Steak

2 tuna steaks (6-9oz. each)
1 Tbs. lemon juice
½ tsp. salt
½ tsp. white pepper

Place skillet on stove set to high and heat 2 minutes. Rub tuna steaks with lemon juice and sprinkle with salt and pepper. Sear steaks in hot skillet 1 or 2 minutes per side (as desired). Serve with stir-fried vegetables.

Garbanzo Bean Salad

1 can (15oz.) garbanzo beans – drained and rinsed
1 medium tomato – chopped
½ medium red onion – diced
6 olives (green or black) - finely sliced
1 Tbs. lemon juice
1 Tbs. lime juice
2 Tbs. parsley
1 tsp. garlic salt
1 tsp. rosemary (optional)

Mix all ingredients together and marinate in refrigerator 15 minutes. Serve cold.

Chapter 7

Choose Right Eating Out

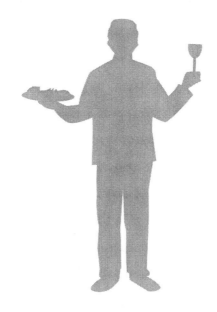

E arlier, we talked about the challenges of eating out in a healthy way. I shared my philosophy about making good choices when you go out to eat and gave you tips on how to curb your appetite. In this chapter, I want to approach the subject of what to eat when you go out.

As I said previously, most food offered in restaurants is unhealthy. So, how can you know the good from the bad? I want you to be fully armed with knowledge, so you can make the best decision possible in every circumstance. In this chapter, I want to take a closer look at the five foods that you should feel safe eating in almost every situation: nuts, seeds, fruits, vegetables, and free range (not grain fed) meat or fish.

You may notice that grain products are not on this list. I've heard people say that cutting grain products from our diets is needless and silly. It is true that for thousands of years people subsisted mainly on grains, but it's also true that those same people had a much higher degree of physical activity, from walking everywhere they went, to planting, harvesting hunting and preparing food. Every daily activity was a physical event. Today, machines wash our clothes, our dishes, sweep our floors, and we simply drive to the grocery down the street for our food. It's also true that throughout history people had a much more limited access to a variety of foods. If it didn't grow where you lived, or if you didn't raise that particular type of animal, there was no way to get that food. Now we live in world where we don't grow our own food, and yet we can eat foods grown all over the world, just by making a quick run to the grocery store. Another startling fact is that people who lived on grain as a staple of their diet didn't live as long as we do. Did you know that grain products and meat that has been fed grain are highly inflammatory, and that chronic inflammation is a contributing factor for most chronic health related illness? Check out Dr. David Seaman's website at www.deflame.com for more information on the harmful effects of inflammation. If you want to trade in your car, grow your own food, and settle for a shorter life, don't let me stop you. If you want to take advantage of what we now know about the human body, health and nutrition, I encourage you to keep reading. I will discuss inflammation in more detail in Chapter 9.

Let's talk about nuts. Nuts are an incredible food. They're really hard-shelled fruits that are high in protein, fiber and good fat (the kind that actually lowers your bad cholesterol). Nuts can be eaten whole, raw, cooked, ground down into flour or made into butter. The only way you should really avoid nuts is when they're covered in salt or candied. There are over 50 different types of nuts, and many varieties of each one. You can add a lot of flavor to your diet by sampling this hearty food. Swap the potato chips on your shopping list for some raw or low sodium roasted nuts. Try a new kind of nut every week for a year. When you go out to eat, look for foods that are cooked with nuts or have nuts added to them, such as pecan crusted baked chicken breast, or salads with almonds or walnuts.

Seeds are actually embryonic plants and many are edible. Seeds have a lot of the same health benefits as nuts, they're rich in fiber, vitamins and protein, but because seeds are smaller, they are sometimes easier to cook and season with. Again, you want to avoid seeds that are covered in salt, but otherwise seeds are extremely good for you. Seeds bring a hearty crunch and unique flavor that enhances many foods. If you see seeds on a menu it's a good sign of a healthy food choice. Another interesting fact is that nuts and seeds are an opposite of grains and are **anti**-inflammatory, actually assisting in ridding your body of inflammation.

Fruits and vegetables are the no-brainer healthy food choice. You don't need me to tell you to eat your vegetables, your mother will be happy to do that for you, but did you know that most restaurants keep fresh fruits and vegetables on hand, even if they aren't on the menu? I mentioned in chapter five that my friend Toby loves the chips at his favorite Mexican restaurant. I like those chips too. In fact, I know that if I eat one, I won't stop. So, when I'm out with friends, and they're all munching on chips and salsa, I'll ask our server for some of the spicy peppers, onions and tomatoes. I can enjoy a healthy snack and not break from my eating plan. Often times, the bar in most restaurants will have celery, olives and cherry tomatoes. I can enjoy an appetizer of carrot sticks or other vegetables instead of eating a deep fried, high fat dish. Fruit is a great desert, and while most restaurants have their fruits covered in sugary syrup, they usually have fresh fruits too. It never hurts to ask if they can bring you a bowl of fresh fruit for dessert. On occasion I have been served a bowl of fresh fruit at a restaurant that was not as sweet as I would like. I will take a single packet of real sugar and sprinkle over it. It sweetens the fruit into a tasty treat and only adds about 14 calories to the dish. Be sure to use real sugar and none of the artificial sweeteners which contain toxic ingredients. Fruits and vegetables are also the perfect side dishes, complementing your main course, rather than saturating your taste buds with salt, fat and oil. Choose a baked potato, steamed veggies or fresh fruit to complement your main dish.

Some people tell me that they can't participate in my healthy food plan because they have to eat meat. I'm always surprised that people think eating healthy means they can't have staple proteins. Most animals are overfed grain-based diets that are highly toxic, from the pesticides used on the grains to the steroids mixed into the feed. Your best choice is to eat free-range, grass-fed meat. You can usually find good quality meat at your local grocery store, but even if you have to look a little harder, the results are worth it, both in taste, and in the healthy quality of the meat. Most fish are now raised on grain-based diets, no different than beef or chicken, that's why I usually look for seafood when I eat out. Most seafood is still caught rather than raised. Taking a little time to know what foods you can eat and why, will empower you when stepping out to eat with friends.

I'll talk more about what to eat later, but right now let me share a few personal examples to give you an idea of how I make healthy choices when eating out. I hardly ever look at menus anymore. They only tempt me to eat the things I know I shouldn't. Instead, when I go out, I ask for custom dishes. For example, if I'm at a steak house, I often have a salad, grilled shrimp and a baked potato. When I order salad, I ask for extra tomato in place of croutons, no cheese, and some fresh citrus fruit on the side, which I squeeze over my salad in place of the dairy-based, high-fat dressing. If fruit isn't available, I opt for a fruit vinaigrette dressing. I order grilled shrimp when it is available, because it is low in calories as well as fat and cholesterol.

As I said before, Mexican food is one of my favorites. When I go out for Mexican food I eat pickled peppers, onions and tomatoes instead of chips. I order a grilled chicken breast with beans and salsa. It has all the flavors I love without the addictive salts and fats, or the inflammatory starches and dairy. You might be wondering if that chicken breast is free range – it probably isn't. But remember, we aren't shooting for perfection. Eating right 90% of the time is what we want to shoot for. We can make a few substitutions without becoming a high-maintenance customer that our friends never want to go out with. Sometimes, the vegetable options at restaurants are cooked in oil or butter. Eating those foods isn't ideal, but it is a *better* choice and remember, eating healthy is all about making the best choice available.

Italian food can be difficult; it's mostly starches and high fat, cheese-based sauces. Not to mention bread, which is a highly inflammatory, addictive food. Luckily, most Italian restaurants now have shrimp-based dishes. I order salad and grilled shrimp, with a side of grilled vegetables. Another great alternative in Italian restaurants is eggplant. Eggplant parmesan is usually battered and fried, but if you ask, most restaurants will grill or bake the eggplant for you. Eggplant is filling and absorbs the flavors it is seasoned with very easily. Here are some great eggplant recipes for you to try at home.

Mediterranean Grilled Eggplant

1 large eggplant
1Tbs. olive oil
3 Tbs. balsamic vinaigrette
1/8 tsp. garlic powder
pinch of thyme, basil and parsley

Heat grill to medium. In a shallow bowl, mix oil, vinaigrette, garlic powder and spices together. Slice eggplant into ½ inch thick slabs. Brush both sides with mix and place on grill. Cook 7-9 minutes on each side.

Baked Eggplant Casserole

1 medium eggplant
1 large tomato
1 medium onion
2 cloves garlic
¼ tsp. thyme

Preheat oven to 375 degrees. Peel and chop eggplant into cubes. Boil eggplant in salted water about 7 minutes. Dice tomato, onion and garlic. Mix tomato, onion, garlic and boiled eggplant in casserole dish and sprinkle with thyme. Bake 45 minutes and serve hot.

Roast Eggplant Salad

1 medium eggplant
1 red onion
1 avocado
1 Tbs. red wine vinegar
1 tsp. Dijon mustard
1 tsp. olive oil
1 pinch salt and pepper
1 lemon
Honey

Preheat oven to 375 degrees. Chop eggplant into 1-inch cubes. Dice onions. Use olive oil to grease cooking sheet. Roast eggplant and onion on cooking sheet 45 minutes, then let cool to room temperature. Peel avocado and dice. Chop cooked eggplant and mix with onions, avocado, red wine vinegar, Dijon mustard, salt and pepper. Zest lemon and add honey to taste. Serve cold.

Southwest Eggplant Stir-fry

1 medium eggplant
1 cup whole kernel corn
1 cup black beans, drained and rinsed
½ cup red pepper, diced
½ cup green onion diced
½ cup cilantro diced
1 Tbs. olive oil
1 Tbs. cumin
1 Tbs. chili powder
1 Tbs. dried parsley
1 tsp. salt
1 tsp. pepper
1 Tbs. onion powder
1 Tbs. garlic salt

Heat grill to medium. Slice eggplant into 1-inch slabs. Sprinkle with garlic salt and onion powder. Grill 15 minutes until tender, then set aside to cool. In wok or sauté pan, heat olive oil, then add red pepper and green onions – stir-fry 2 minutes. Dice eggplant and add to wok with corn, beans, cilantro, chili powder, cumin, salt, pepper and parsley. Stir-fry 5 minutes and serve hot.

Indian Spiced Eggplant and Cauliflower Stew

2 Tbs. curry powder
1 tsp. mustard seeds
1 Tbs. olive oil
1 large onion sliced
2 cloves garlic - minced
1 tsp. fresh ginger - grated
¾ tsp. salt
1 medium eggplant, cut into 1-inch cubes
3 cups cauliflower florets
2 cups diced tomatoes
1 can (15 oz.) chickpeas - rinsed
½ cup water

In large pot, toast curry powder and mustard seeds approximately 1 minute. Remove to a bowl. In same pot, heat oil and cook onions, garlic and ginger with salt 3 to 4 minutes until onion is tender. Add eggplant, cauliflower, tomatoes, chickpeas, curry powder, mustard seeds and water. Bring to a simmer, cover and reduce heat. Cook 15 minutes or until vegetables are tender.

Chapter 8

Unlocking Food Addiction

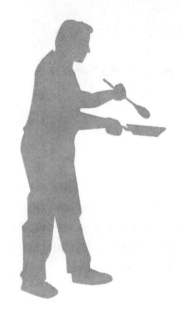

M any studies and research projects are being conducted to discover if food is really addictive. For those of us who have struggled with weight issues we know the power of food. The American Psychiatric Association's Diagnostic and Statistical Manual of Mental Disorders says that addiction is characterized by three or more of the following: "tolerance, withdrawal, large amounts over a long period, unsuccessful efforts to cut down, time spent in obtaining the substance replaces social, occupational, or recreational activities, continued use causes adverse consequences." It seems pretty clear that for many people, food is an addiction, but let's takes a closer look at the science of food addiction to see if there are any keys to break food's hold over us.

Recent studies at Princeton and the University of Florida have shown the addictive nature of refined foods – salt, fats and sugars[1]. Researches fed rats a diet of highly refined foods. Wouldn't you know it, those rats got fat. What's really fascinating is the addictive nature of the refined food diet. It actually affects your body chemistry in the same way narcotics do. Here's the story...

The rats didn't just get fat; they got hooked on the junk food. Basically, they offered the rats two food options, the normal rat food the animals had lived on their whole lives, or a new food that was highly refined, much like the food most Americans eat on a regular basis. The rats loved the junk food and wouldn't stop eating it. It seemed the more junk the rats ate, the more they wanted to eat. When the scientists took away the highly refined food option, the rats went on a hunger strike. They actually refused to eat rather than eat their normal rat food without the salt, fat and sugar. Consider what that says about what we eat. The scientists even gave the rats mild electrical shocks in their feet when they ate the highly refined foods, but just like an alcoholic or drug addict, the rats endured the pain to get those foods rather than eat the healthy food.

The studies also revealed that the rats eating the refined food diet gained more weight than rats fed a diet high in unrefined fats. And when

---

1 "Junkie Food." NewScientist 4 Sept. 2010: 38-41 & "Junk Food Turns Rats Into Addicts" Science News 21 Nov. 2009: Vol. 176 #11

the rats were taken off the refined diet, they lost weight much more slowly than their fat counterparts that had not been on the refined diet. Sound familiar? These rats got so addicted to the refined foods that they would rather starve than eat healthy food. They were so hooked. They couldn't stop eating the junk food. They gained weight fast and couldn't get it off. It sounds like the story of my life.

When the study was over, the scientists looked into the chemistry of the rats' brains and digestive systems. What they found was that the refined foods actually altered the rats' body chemistry. Eating the refined foods released a chemical called dopamine, which is normally produced during pleasurable circumstances. For the rats, the dopamine was like cocaine, they wanted it all the time. But just like drugs, the more they ate the refined food diet forcing their bodies to produce dopamine, the more junk food they needed to feel that same level of pleasure.

Many of us have responded to food just like the rats did, but we don't have too. We may have the same bio-chemical reaction to refined food, we may be just as addicted and have the same weight issues, but we aren't controlled by instinct. We have the God-given ability of reason and self will, so we can choose to say no to our body's urges and cravings. Our strength lies in knowing what is happening to us and why we want those foods that are so unhealthy.

Take a moment to think about your life. Do you tend to overeat or crave food when you're stressed, scared or unhappy? Do you feel like food is the one thing you can give yourself as much as you want? Do you celebrate with food, comfort with food, go looking for food when you're bored? These are all signs that you are responding to your body's chemical response to the food, not the food itself. Food alone cannot make you happy. Sure, if you don't have food it may be all you think about, but the body's natural desire for food is to give you energy, not to make you happy.

Think of your body like a car. A car needs gas to fuel it, without gas the car won't go. We go to a gas station to fill the car's gas tank, which is a specially designed compartment made to store a reasonable amount of fuel. We wouldn't dream of going on a long trip with only a few gallons in the tank. Neither would we want to fill the interior of our car with portable gas cans. In fact, carrying gasoline anywhere in your car except the gas tank is extremely dangerous. Now, if we lived in the middle of the dessert, hundreds of miles from the nearest gas station, we might desire to keep additional gas with us all the time. But most of us live a few minutes away from the nearest convenience store. It is reckless to risk our safety and the safety of those who might be riding with us by carrying excess gas.

Our bodies need food much the same way a car needs gas. And our body has a natural reaction to the surplus of food we take in, it gets stored as fat to be used in case we can't get food as often as we need it. But just like excess fuel in a car, too much fat on our bodies is dangerous. It strains our circulatory system, our joints, frame and spine. It stores toxins in our bodies because we consume more than our liver can filter. It robs us of energy because our digestive system is constantly processing the food we ingest. We live in a world where food is common, not scarce. We need to give our body only what it needs, and not place other demands on it.

So how do we find relief from food addiction? I want to talk about two very important areas that we need to work on to break our addiction from food. First is the food itself, and the fact that some foods are addictive and others aren't. Then we need to see what drives us to turn to food when we aren't hungry, the psychological issues that push us toward food addiction.

I've said this before but it's worth saying again: we can't stop eating, but we can stop eating addictive foods. You may not be able to stop eating at just one potato chip. The salt and refined fat in the chips fire false signals in your brain and body chemistry that make you want to eat until you're sick. But whole foods are not addictive. I've never heard anyone say I had some spinach and just couldn't stop eating. People assume that it's because whole foods don't taste good, but that simply isn't true. Whole foods just don't affect your body chemistry the way refined foods do. Chiropractic care is based on the theory that your body is made to be healthy, and if given the time and care it needs, most physical problems can be healed naturally. Before the technological age, the study of medicine was much closer to Chiropractic care. Natural plants and minerals were used to assist the body in its natural healing processes. Modern medicine introduced synthetically produced chemicals that stimulate, manipulate and force the body into a desired state. Most chemicals work by causing a negative reaction in the body. Refined foods are much like the synthetic chemicals used in medicine that have a real and lasting impact on the natural function of our bodies. Have you noticed drug commercials on television and the long list of negative side effects? Some of the side effects sound worse than the problem they claim to treat! Refined foods should come with a list of the negative side effects caused by eating them. Whole foods on the other hand support the natural process of health and offer the building blocks required for the body to be healthy with no negative side effects.

The only way to break the addiction of refined foods is to fast from them. That is one purpose of the 7-Day Cleanse. In most cases, a week is very effective in breaking the addiction to refined foods. After breaking the addiction, some people have the will power to be able to splurge without falling back into addiction. Most of us on the other hand, myself included, need help to break the addiction cycle when it comes to food. By sticking closely to a whole food diet, we begin to return our body chemistry back to a natural state. I really can't say enough about the power of whole foods. They give us the fuel we need to tackle the issues we face each day and help us to stay healthy. Almost every disease known to man is affected by our diet, from epilepsy, to cancer and heart disease.

God had a really great plan when He created food. All of the foods that we consider whole foods, foods that are in their natural state the way God gave them to us, the way they grow out of the ground, on the tree, in nature, are foods that have all the nutrients packed within to support our health and fight disease. Whole foods are also low in calories so we can eat virtually all we want of them and never get fat. The foods we have created with all our "wisdom" are foods robbed of nutrition, highly inflammatory and high in calories. We are eating the very things that are making us sick and fat.

There is another aspect of food addiction that should also be noted and that is the emotional side. According to www.Addictions.org, a website dedicated to helping people overcome addictive behaviors, most people who struggle with food addiction fall into a similar personality profile: *They are often people pleasers who tend to hide their real feelings. They struggle with low self-esteem and poor body image...*[2] For most people, food addiction begins at a young age when food is seen as a remedy or comfort to problems and stress. The way you view yourself is equally as important as what you eat. You need to know and believe that you can lose weight. You also need to accept the truth that food does not make you happy. That doesn't mean that food isn't enjoyable, but eating doesn't lead to happiness. If you feel that food is your escape or your reward for enduring something you don't like, that is an emotional issue that needs to be explored and healed.

I meet people every day who feel trapped and defeated by food. They are sick in body and spirit because of the weight they can't seem be get rid of. If you feel you are trapped and defeated, my passion is to help you, through knowledge and the power that comes from taking responsibility for your choices, to see that you can be healthy and lose weight. It's not an impossible task, and you are not hopeless, but you have to take control of your life. You are not a rat in a cage, ruled by your body's impulses. You are a person made in the image of God and given the freedom to choose your own actions. Food addiction is real, and refined foods really do affect the way you think and feel about food. But you can change; you can start today even if you've tried a hundred times and failed. You can be successful.

Following are some recipes that are simply delicious. Take the time to see how great whole foods can make you feel. This isn't an impossible plan,

---

2 http://info.addictions.org/index/Addictive+Behaviors/Overeating

and it will change your life. If you want to be healthy, it starts with breaking the addiction and giving yourself permission to succeed.

Warm Spinach Salad

2 cups baby spinach
1 can tuna (2.5oz.)
1 Tbs lemon juice
½ tsp. garlic powder
1/8 tsp. salt
1/8 tsp. pepper

Mix lemon juice, garlic powder, salt and pepper. Microwave 30 seconds. Drizzle over spinach and top with tuna.

Sautéed Vegetables with Cashews

½ cup chicken or vegetable broth
1 cup onion – chopped
1 cup red pepper – chopped
1 cup yellow pepper – chopped
1 cup yellow squash – chopped
1 cup zucchini – chopped
1 cup snow peas
¼ cup cashews – chopped

In large pot, heat broth until steaming. Add onion, peppers, squash and zucchini. Cover and simmer 5 minutes. Add snow peas and cover, simmer another 2 minutes. Drain remaining broth and mix in cashews. Serve hot.

Arugula Salad with Walnuts

½ medium onion – thinly sliced
1 cup hot water
2 Tbs. vinegar
1 bunch arugula
1 Tbs. garlic salt
2 Tbs. parsley
1 Tbs. lemon juice
½ cup walnuts – chopped

Let onions soak in hot water and vinegar at least 5 minutes. Mix garlic salt, parsley and lemon juice together. Mix arugula and onions together and drizzle with juice mix. Toss with walnuts and serve.

Fresh Avocado Salad

1 head romaine lettuce – outer leaves discarded, then chopped
1 large tomato – seeded and diced
1 small red pepper – julienned
½ medium avocado – finely chopped
2 Tbs. sesame or sunflower seeds – optional
2 tsp. lemon juice
2 tsp. balsamic vinegar
Olive oil to taste
Salt and pepper to taste

Cut off the bottoms of the romaine leaves and discard. Chop the romaine and toss with tomato, red pepper, avocado and nuts. Mix lemon juice, balsamic vinegar and olive oil to taste. Drizzle dressing over salad and enjoy.

Creamy Squash Soup

1 medium butternut squash – peeled and cubed (1 inch cubes)
1 large onion - diced
3 cloves garlic – minced
1 Tbs. ginger – minced
1 tsp. turmeric
1 tsp. curry powder
3 cups chicken or vegetable broth
1 can coconut milk (6oz.)
½ cup cilantro – chopped
1 pinch salt
1 pinch pepper

Sauté onion in large pan with 1 tablespoon chicken or vegetable broth about 5 minutes, stirring frequently. Add garlic and ginger, continue cooking 1 minute. Add turmeric and curry powder, mix well, then add remaining broth and squash. Bring to boil, then reduce heat and simmer 10 minutes. Remove from heat and allow to cool. Mix with coconut milk and blend 1 minute (you'll need to blend the soup in batches). Return soup to pan and reheat to serve. Mix in salt and pepper, and top with cilantro.

Chapter 9

Dietary Inflammation

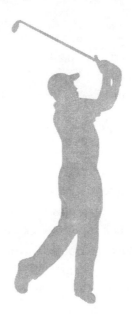

W e've talked a lot about what we should eat and should not eat. But now, I want to go into more detail about *why* eating some foods are so bad for you. Everyone knows that fatty foods make us fat, and we've discussed the addictive nature of refined foods. You also need to know about dietary inflammation, why it's harmful for you, and what to do to avoid it.

Inflammation is a nonspecific immune response. Most of us think of inflammation in the context of an injury. A very simple explanation for how inflammation works to assist the body when it is injured is this. When we stress our body, say we sprain our ankle, the ligaments and tendons in our ankle get stretched, causing tiny breaks and tears that need to be repaired, so our body goes into healing mode. Basically, our immune system sends in the National Guard to help. Blood filled with healing agents surrounds the area. This results in swelling and pain for us, but it is our body's way of healing. Pain tells us that something is wrong and attention is required. It also warns us to stop using that part of our body for awhile. In this case, the pain would alert us that damage has taken place in our ankle and tell us to not put weight on that injured leg until it is well. That is an inflammatory response, and it is a positive response, because it causes care for our injury. When we have a physical injury, we need inflammation to help us heal.

We can also have stress injuries when we do something that slowly weakens and eventually wears down our body. Consider a mechanic who is constantly bent over the engine of a car, putting strain on his lower back and legs. Over time, the muscles and tendons get weak and start to function improperly. Our body will send in the troops to see about fixing that area, which results in inflammation. The mechanic suffers from chronic back, hip and leg pain, but it is actually a result of his body trying to heal.

There is yet a third way that inflammation affects us, it's called dietary inflammation. Certain foods actually cause our body to respond as if it were injured. It isn't inflammation akin to an injury; your body doesn't send in all the troops and flood a specific area with blood. It's similar to the government raising the terrorist threat level and security measures are stepped up everywhere. It may not seem like such a bad thing, especially since you don't usually feel it or notice when it is happening, but dietary inflammation leads to chronic inflammation. This is inflammation at the cellular level which in turn leads to major diseases such as cancer, heart disease, Alzheimer's disease, Multiple Sclerosis and Parkinson's disease, just to name a few. Chronic inflammation can leave you feeling tired and unwell, aches and pains, acne and arthritis and other symptoms. The main causes of chronic inflammation are a diet of processed foods including dairy and grain products, stress, and lack of exercise.

Dietary inflammation is being studied with more and more information learned every day. Most of us know that diets high in cholesterol and fat can lead to heart and circulatory disease. Imagine combining that poor diet with a diet of foods that cause chronic inflammation? It's a recipe for disaster. I not only want people to understand that eating whole foods is a great way to lose weight and enjoy a healthy life, but also to know the dangers of eating foods that cause them harm. We can reverse this harmful effect our diets are having on our bodies. We just need to know how.

So how does dietary inflammation injure us? Consider again the comparison to the raised security levels our nation faces as we try to protect ourselves from harm. Imagine what your life would be like if you had to deal with troops on the streets, security checks at public buildings, and constant inspections. At first you might feel reassured, but as time went by you might begin to feel harassed, frustrated, and even resentful. You would probably curb your activities to avoid all the red tape you encountered every time you went out. You might even work less to avoid the constant scrutiny. You might consider that doing the normal things of life just weren't worth the hassle. Now imagine how you might feel as constant warnings about terrorist attacks went by with no visible danger? You might grow skeptical about the danger and not take the warnings seriously.

That is exactly what happens to your body. The immune system slows, your joints lose their elasticity, and your body does less and less as it conserves itself and avoids the difficulties arising from the constant inflammation. Most people deal with these issues by taking medicines, which only mask the problem. Anti-inflammatory drugs work by inhibiting the production of prostaglandin E2 (PGE2), which is a hormone that affects the contraction and relaxation of smooth muscle, the dilation and constriction of blood vessels, control of blood pressure, and modulation of inflammation. PGE2 is released from the walls of blood vessels in response to infection or inflammation and affects the brain by activating the "fever response." This is good. That is a part of the healing response. But, it is also a potent stimulator of pain and causes the breakdown of cartilage and bone and can promote cancer, heart disease and Alzheimer's disease among other things. It's one of those things that are good for you unless your body is over producing it. Not unlike so many things in life, a little bit of some things is good, a lot can be bad. Too many troops on the street usually lead to a loss of freedom and a rise in the corruption of authority.

So, while your body needs the inflammatory response and PGE2 for healing, too much can hurt you. So where does all this PGE2 come from? PGE2 is produced from Omega-6 fatty acids found in all grains, cereals and flour products. It's in most packaged foods and cooking oils. It's also in the meat of animals that are fed high-grain diets. When we eat these foods we are causing the very problems that plague us and keep us from feeling like doing the things we need to do to lose weight. Let's face it, if you feel achy, tired and stiff from dietary inflammation you aren't going to feel like exercising or doing anything active. It's a vicious cycle.

How do we stop chronic inflammation? The good news is that following my new Chose Right, Eat Right, and Move Right plan, discussed in depth in *I Don't Go With Fat Boys*, you will actually eliminate the dietary inflammation that leads to chronic inflammation. By choosing right, you can actually eat your way to rid your body of the contaminants that are producing the inflammation. As your body returns to a healthy state, you will feel more energized, less achy and stiff. Moving Right, and getting active doesn't seem impossible for you anymore, and exercise is a great stress reducer. The way we stop inflammation is through eating a whole food diet. Fruits and vegetables are full of anti-inflammatory Omega-3 fatty acids. Eating healthy foods will help you lose weight, but they also produce optimal conditions for our bodies to work the way they were designed to work.

I have a friend who loves to play golf, but he often finds his ball buried in the deep grass around the greens. His golf club, which is designed to get the ball up into the air for a soft landing near the hole, was great when his ball was on the short grass of the fairway, but too often his ball was in tall, thick grass, which kept his club from operating as it was designed. There are different ways to deal with such a problem, the first and most effective is to figure out why he was hitting so many errant shots that missed the green and landed in the rough grass. My friend chose a quicker method. He actually ground down the edge of his club so that it was like a blade cutting through the grass. Because he plays golf as a hobby and doesn't compete in tournaments, he wasn't concerned with the fact that his club was no longer regulation and was basically breaking the rules. We often view our lives the same way. We recognize that we are overweight and need to make changes for our health, so that we can look and feel better, but the cost of changing our diet and living a healthy lifestyle seems too difficult. We prefer a quick fix despite the cost. Chronic inflammation is a proven concern, but many people would rather take a pill for the symptoms than change their diet. Oddly enough, the food they eat is making the medications ineffective.

Here are some fast and delicious recipes, high in Omega-3 fatty acids that will help your body balance into a more natural state of wellness. Don't believe the myth that eating healthy is too hard and can't taste good. Give these recipes a shot and you'll be surprised at the results.

Huevos Rancheros

2 free range eggs
½ cup black beans – drained, rinsed and mashed
1 tsp. lime juice
½ cup chopped cilantro
¼ cup salsa

Bring a pot of water to a slow simmer, and adjust heat to maintain a consistent water temperature. Crack open eggs directly into the hot water and cook 5 minutes. While the eggs are cooking place beans in a skillet and heat. Add lime juice, salt and pepper (for a spicier meal add a dash of cayenne pepper) and stir. Spread beans on plate, place poached eggs on top of the beans, sprinkle cilantro over all and top with salsa.

Black Pepper Salmon with Fennel

1 ½ pounds salmon – quartered
1 large fennel bulb – sliced thin
¼ cup chicken or vegetable broth
¼ tsp salt
1 tsp black pepper
1 Tbs. lemon juice

Rub salmon with 1 Tbs. lemon juice then sprinkle with salt and pepper. Set aside. In medium pan stir-fry fennel with about 1 Tbs. of broth approximately 1 minute. Add the remainder of the broth and lemon juice, place salmon on top. Turn heat to low and cover, cook approximately 5 minutes.

Mustard Dill Salmon with Cauliflower

1 ½ pounds salmon – quartered
4 cups cauliflower florets
4 Tbs. dill
1 Tbs. Dijon mustard
1 Tbs. honey
1 Tbs. lemon juice
¼ tsp. salt
¼ tsp. pepper

Bring water in steamer to boil. Steam cauliflower approximately 5 minutes until tender. Remove cauliflower from basket. Rub salmon with lemon juice and steam in the same basket as the cauliflower approximately 4 minutes. Mix mustard, honey, dill, salt and pepper together to make sauce (if flavor is too strong dilute with water). Drizzle sauce over salmon and cauliflower.

Tuna Salad with Walnuts

2 cans light tuna
¼ cup celery - diced
¼ cup white onion – diced
3 Tbs. walnuts - chopped
3 Tbs. parsley
1 head Romaine – outer leaves removed
6 cherry tomatoes – quartered
¼ cup sunflower seeds
1 Tbs. Dijon mustard
1 tsp. honey
½ tsp garlic powder
3 Tbs. lemon juice
½ tsp Italian herbs
¼ cup water

Cut off the bottoms of the romaine leaves and discard. Chop Romaine and mix with tuna, onions, celery, walnuts, cherry tomatoes and parsley. In a separate container, mix sunflower seeds with mustard, honey, garlic powder, lemon juice, herbs and water. Toss with salad and serve.

Southwest Scramble

3 free range eggs
½ cup red pepper – diced
½ cup yellow pepper – diced
½ cup green onion – diced
1 jalapeno pepper – seeded and diced
1 Tbs. olive oil

Sauté peppers and onion in olive oil until tender, about 4 minutes. Crack eggs and whisk until well mixed. Pour eggs into sauté pan and stir. Cook additional 4 minutes, sprinkle with salt and pepper.

Chapter 10

Stocking Your Pantry

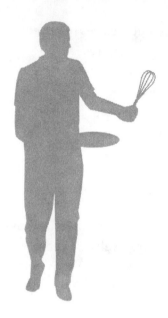

We've covered a lot of ground and talked about dealing with issues that arise from trying to eat right. Armed with the right knowledge and the power of choice, we really can lose weight and get healthy. So why do so many people fail? I think one of the biggest reasons we fail is because even though we know the right things to do, and we really want to make lasting changes, we all get tired and want to take the easiest path to rest and relaxation. Face it, at the end of a long day, you've worked hard and now you look forward to getting home and reading a good book or watching your favorite television show. The thought of preparing a healthy meal sometimes seems daunting. It feels like in that moment it would be so much easier to just grab a hamburger on the way home, not to mention you may be craving some comfort food. That's an easy way to fall off the healthy lifestyle wagon. When you get home and open the pantry or refrigerator and what you see are healthy foods that need preparation but all you've got the energy for is sticking something in the microwave, you lose your determination to stay with your healthy plan. I want to help you have options; delicious, easy, healthy meal options whenever it's time to eat. Let's start with the basics, some of the most common utensils you'll need to keep in your kitchen.

First, if you're going to eat healthy, you'll need a good chopping block. Almost every meal you prepare will need vegetables and a good place to cut, peel, remove seeds and slice is essential. There's nothing more frustrating than trying to cut vegetables on a plate or in a space that's too small. So get a good cutting board, one that you can wash easily and give it a prime place in your kitchen. A good set of sharp knives nearby will complement your board and will make preparing delicious, healthy meals much easier.

Second, you'll want a supply of good freezer bags. Many times a recipe will call for a portion of something, like a half a cup of red pepper diced. A portion of the pepper is left. Go ahead and dice the entire pepper, then put the unused portion into a freezer bag. Keep a permanent marker nearby to label your freezer bags and soon you'll have a stock of ingredients ready to be used without any preparation. Good freezer bags will save you a lot of time and money.

Another indispensable item is a hand held strainer. You don't need a large colander to drain a can of vegetables and just using the lid of a can won't help you when rinsing the fruit or vegetables. A nice, hand held strainer will be very useful, especially if you are pressed for time and using a lot of canned goods to make your meal. A small strainer can be washed off easily or thrown into the dishwasher, and allows you to use canned foods without the sugary syrups or metallic taste you sometimes get from the can.

Finally, make sure you have a few good pots and pans for cooking. Buying a boxed set can be an inexpensive way to acquire a set with a variety of sizes, but a good cook knows that one well-made pan is worth four poorly made ones. You should look for pans that have a flat bottom. I know that all pans should be flat on bottom, but metal often warps, especially if isn't made with good materials and taken care of. Many cookware companies use cheap materials. The result is an unlevel pan that won't heat evenly. When you shop, take a ruler or other straight edge device that will allow you to see if the pan is well made. When you finish cooking with your pans, let them set and cool rather than dousing them in water, which can warp the metal.

Now let's talk about what to keep in your refrigerator. Most homes have mustard and ketchup in the fridge, but what should you have on hand to help you stick to your health goals? First, you should clean out the refrigerator. If you're a neat person who likes things clean in the kitchen then you're ahead of the game. If you're like most people, you may have food in your refrigerator that is weeks old. Take a day and get all the junk out. Even if you aren't eating junk food anymore and the only thing left in your refrigerator is a pizza box that's three weeks old, just seeing it every day will make it harder to let go of the refined, addictive foods. When your refrigerator is clean and bright, with everything neatly organized, you'll want to keep it that way and getting in it to get healthy foods will be encouraging.

Next, you always need fresh vegetables, so take your time when you shop. Look for the things that catch your eye, even if you've never eaten them before. The internet is full of cooking tips and recipes. If you want to experiment with food, vegetables are the way to go. Keep them clean and fresh in your refrigerator so that meal times don't become chores. When you feel hungry, a salad is always an easy and healthy meal or snack, so keep your favorite lettuce on hand, along with any extra veggies that you like with your salad. Cherry tomatoes are a quick and easy salad add-on, and they give your dishes flavor, color and juiciness.

Another thing you'll need to keep in your refrigerator is meat. Unless you're a vegetarian, you'll want to have meat on hand. Finding good, grass fed beef or lamb or free-range chicken is essential to success. You'll want to keep some meat on hand to enhance your meals. Meat doesn't last as long as most vegetables, but keeping some in your refrigerator will help you stick to your guns when the junk food cravings come calling.

Fresh fruits or vegetable juice is another handy thing to keep in the fridge. Water is the nectar of life, but everyone loves some flavor occasionally; an added splash of fruit juice in water is a great way to get it. Soda is loaded with sugar and is highly addictive with almost zero nutrient value. Beware of prepackaged juices, they're pasteurized and tainted with chemical preservatives. Likewise cocktail juices are usually highly sweetened with sugar or corn syrups and can be just as bad as sodas. Another great drink is water flavored with slices of fruit or even cucumber or mint. A pitcher can last all day and cost almost nothing to keep around.

Chicken or vegetable broth is also an indispensable item to keep on hand. Many recipes call for broth to give them flavor. And broth is also a great substitute for oil when it comes to sautéing. A little broth heated in a skillet will work great for cooking vegetables and seafood quickly while giving them a wonderful flavor. You can make your own broth if you have a pressure cooker or large stock pot, but organic broth can easily be found at your supermarket. If you're buying broth, look for low sodium and watch out for chemical preservatives. A good broth will make cooking great meals fast and easy.

Finally, you'll want to keep some free-range fresh eggs in the refrigerator. A lot of recipes call for eggs and they're a great source of Omega-3 fatty acid and protein that lasts longer than meat. Eggs are easy to prepare and can be cooked in many different ways that produce unique flavors. You can often find farm-raised eggs at your local farmer's market if your grocery store doesn't carry them.

Freezers make eating healthy a breeze. While we want to eat fresh foods as often as possible, keeping a good supply of foods in your freezer will really be a benefit when you're in a hurry or don't have the energy to prepare everything from scratch. Microwaves make defrosting and steaming from frozen a breeze, so let's take at look at few things you should keep on hand in your freezer.

Frozen vegetables are a must have if you're going to maintain a healthy diet. Frozen vegetables may not be as flavorful as fresh veggies, but when it comes to convenience the trade off is even. You can buy a large assortment of vegetables from the frozen food isle at your local supermarket. They're easy to cook from frozen in the microwave. Frozen vegetables can make a quick and easy side dish, or with a good sauce be a great centerpiece meal. You can also add them easily to soups, stews or casseroles to increase the nutrient value of your meal.

Frozen seafood is a great way to keep delicious food at your fingertips. Most seafood can be thawed in just a few minutes either in running water or a water bath. Shrimp is my favorite and it's becoming less expensive every day. Watch out for farm raised fish, which are usually fed a grain-based diet and can be inflammatory. Crab meat is also a good choice and can enhance many dishes while keeping them light and delicious.

Frozen sauce is also a great way to make meal preparation a breeze. Prepackaged sauces are usually high in preservatives and refined fats and sugars. If you can take some time, perhaps one day a month and prepare delicious sauces made from fresh ingredients, you can bag portion sizes and freeze them. When you're ready to make your meal, the sauce will thaw as the other ingredients cook, and in just a few minutes your sauce will be heated through and delicious, making your meal rich and flavorful.

Finally, let's talk about what dry goods to keep on hand. You'll need a good stock of spices and herbs. Spices and herbs add zest and flavor to any meal. The right seasonings make an average meal outstanding. If you don't have a good supply of spices you can buy some racks with a good variety included. I remember in college eating at the cafeteria the food was often so bland everyone used salt and pepper to give their food flavor. But food that is well cooked doesn't have to have a huge dose of salt. In fact, food that is well seasoned may not need any salt at all. Experiment until you find a good set of spices and herbs that you really enjoy. Spices and herbs are cheap, add tons of flavor and no calories.

Beans are a great source of fiber, protein and iron. You can cook them in a myriad of ways and the best part is they're very inexpensive. They also last a long time. The one drawback to beans is that they often require a lengthy cooking time. If you're organized, you can get beans going in a slow cooker before you leave for work and find them ready to eat with when you get home. If you need beans in a hurry, you can use canned beans. When you buy canned beans or any canned vegetable, look at the ingredients to make sure you are getting food without chemicals or preservatives added. When you use canned beans, strain the juices and rinse them to get the cleanest and best flavors and add your favorite seasoning for enhanced flavor.

Although you'll want to use fresh foods as often as possible, canned goods are a good compromise when time is short. Canned vegetables are a third resort after fresh or frozen, but in the right circumstance they may be the best choice. A good variety of canned fruits and vegetables can go a long way toward making a meal enjoyable. Canned goods also keep a very long time, so consider your canned goods insurance against bad food choices. It's easier to open a can of fruit or vegetables than have to restart your eating plan. You can also get some canned or packaged fish, especially smoked salmon or tuna to give any meal a unique flavor and added protein without adding a lot of calories.

We want to stay away from packaged foods because they are often full of refined fats, salt and sweeteners, but there are some packaged foods that are healthier alternatives to most of the foods found on grocery store shelves. Look for gourmet or organic brands, they may cost a bit more, but these foods shouldn't be the main source of your meals, and spending a little extra to stay healthy is well worth the cost. Some well selected prepackaged foods can make a great base to be beefed up with fresh or frozen vegetables and spiced up with your dried herbs and spices to make a delicious and filling meal. Keeping a variety of spice packages on hand for quick meal preparation is a good plan. Make sure to check the packaging and chose those with nothing but natural spices, no chemicals added. Gourmet soups are a great way to prepare a really delicious meal fast. Organic sauces can also be found that will add flavor to ordinary meals that would otherwise be bland. Make it fun. Search your grocery store and look for surprising alternatives to the prepackaged, processed foods of your past.

Keeping good foods in your home is the best way to avoid getting caught with fast food cravings. Here are few more recipes to keep you eating healthy.

Orange Stir Fry Sauce

1 cup frozen orange juice concentrate
2 Tbs. apple sauce
1 tsp. vinegar
½ Tbs. minced garlic
½ Tbs. minced ginger
1 Tbs. low sodium soy sauce

Heat saucepan over medium heat. Add applesauce, garlic and ginger. Cook 1 minute, stirring constantly. Add orange juice concentrate, vinegar and soy sauce. Simmer over low heat, stirring frequently until sauce reduces. Serve over steamed vegetables or use in stir fry.

Mint Salsa (great with seafood)

1 Tbs. mint - finely chopped
1 Tbs. cilantro - finely chopped
1 Tbs. scallion - finely chopped
1 tsp. ginger - minced
1 medium tomato – seeded and finely chopped
3 cloves garlic – pressed
3 Tbs. lemon juice
salt and pepper to taste

Mix all ingredients together and chill. Serve cold over salmon, tuna, or other seafood.

Tomato Salsa

1 large tomato, seeded and finely diced
3 Tbs. onion – minced
3 cloves garlic – pressed
2 Tbs. jalapeno – minced and seeded
1 Tbs. ginger – minced
1 Tbs. pumpkin seeds – chopped
1 cup cilantro – chopped
2 Tbs. lime juice
salt and pepper to taste

For chunky salsa, simply mix all ingredients together. Chill half an hour to allow flavors to mingle before serving. You can also put all ingredients in a food processor, blend approximately 1 minute and then chill. Eat with raw vegetables or it is great poured over steaming hot vegetables or baked potato for a great south of the border flavor.

Chunky Avocado Salsa

6 cloves garlic – pressed
¼ cup scallions – minced
2 jalapenos – seeded and minced
1 cup cilantro - chopped
8 cherry tomatos – quartered
1 medium avocado – cubed
¼ cup lime juice
salt and pepper to taste

In a large bowl mix all ingredients and drizzle with lime juice. Toss lightly and serve with any raw or cold vegetable

Fresh Marinara Sauce

1 large tomato – finely diced
4 cloves garlic – minced
1 large can tomato paste (12oz.)
1 ¼ tsp. oregano
¼ tsp. salt
¼ tsp. pepper
1/3 cup parsley
2 tsp. chicken or vegetable broth
1 tsp. cooking wine

In medium saucepan heat broth over medium-high heat. Sauté garlic 1 minute. Add tomato paste, tomatoes, oregano, salt, pepper and wine. Bring to simmer, then reduce heat and cook 20 minutes. Stir in parsley and serve over baked eggplant thickly sliced

Avocado-Mango Crab Salad

1 medium avocado diced
1 medium mango diced
½ pound chopped crab meat
1 head of romaine lettuce torn into bite sized pieces
Juice of ½ medium lime
Black pepper to taste

Mix all ingredients in a mixing bowl. Serve in single serving salad bowls.

Conclusion

Ok, I've told you my story and shown you that, whether you have struggled for just a few years or for your entire life as I have, there is an answer to your weight problem. I hope you gained some helpful information and that you will choose to start your own journey toward your health goals. This is not the only answer, but it is the one that works for me. I am 80 pounds lighter with lower cholesterol, triglycerides and blood pressure because of this lifestyle plan. If this former "fat boy" can do it, you can too. And, on the days you struggle or fall, know that is normal, and tomorrow is another day. When there are days you just can't get it right, know that we have all been there, that's real life. The only way you will not be successful is if you stop trying. At any moment in time, the very next thing you put into your mouth can be a healthy choice. I have failed a thousand times, but keeping on with it I am 80 pounds lighter, and still on my way down.

Whew! The book is finished. I think I will go celebrate with a pint of Chunky Monkey. Oops, I meant to say carrot sticks and fruit didn't I?

Dr. Fuhrman's Micronutrient Scores

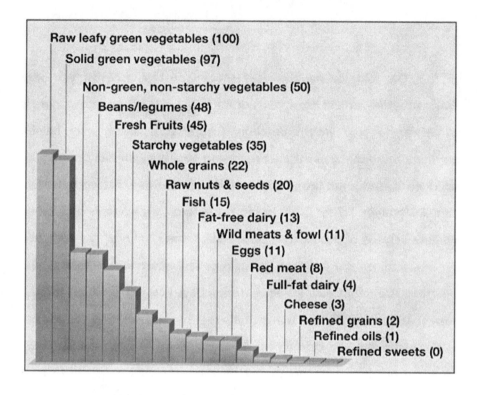

Raw leafy green vegetables (100)
Solid green vegetables (97)
Non-green, non-starchy vegetables (50)
Beans/legumes (48)
Fresh Fruits (45)
Starchy vegetables (35)
Whole grains (22)
Raw nuts & seeds (20)
Fish (15)
Fat-free dairy (13)
Wild meats & fowl (11)
Eggs (11)
Red meat (8)
Full-fat dairy (4)
Cheese (3)
Refined grains (2)
Refined oils (1)
Refined sweets (0)

Nutrient Density

Nutrient Density is a critical concept in devising and recommending dietary and nutritional advice to patients and to the public. Not merely vitamins and minerals, but adequate consumption of phytochemicals is essential for proper functioning of the immune system and to enable our body's detoxification and cellular repair mechanisms that protect us from chronic diseases.

Nutritional science in the last twenty years has demonstrated that colorful plant foods contain a huge assortment of protective compounds, most of which still remain unnamed. Only by eating an assortment of nutrient-rich natural foods can we access these protective compounds and prevent the common diseases that afflict Americans. Our modern, low-nutrient eating style has led to an overweight population, the majority of whom develop diseases of nutritional ignorance, causing our medical costs to spiral out of control.

To guide people toward the most nutrient dense foods, I developed a 0-100 scale of micronutrient scores called the Nutrient Density Line, which ranks categories of foods based on their ratio of nutrients to calories.

Because phytochemicals are largely unnamed and unmeasured, these rankings underestimate the healthful properties of colorful natural plant foods compared to processed foods and animal products. One thing we do know is that the foods that contain the highest amount of known nutrients are the same foods that contain the most unknown nutrients too. So even though these rankings may not consider the phytochemical number sufficiently they are still a reasonable measurement of phytochemical content.

Keep in mind that nutrient density scoring is not the only factor that determines good health. For example, if we only ate foods with a high nutrient density score our diet would be too low in fat. So we have to pick some foods with lower nutrient density scores (but preferably the healthier ones) to include in our high nutrient diet. Additionally, if a slim or highly physically active individual ate only the highest nutrient foods they would become so full from all of the fiber and nutrients that they would not be able to meet their caloric needs, and they would eventually become too thin. This of course gives you a hint at the secret to permanent weight control – eat the greatest quantity of the foods with the highest micronutrient scores, and lesser amounts of foods with lower scores. For more information on the Nutrient Density Line, please refer to *Eat to Live* (2011 edition), pages 118-122.

This information taken from Dr. Joel Fuhrman's website:

http://drfuhrman.com/library/article17.aspx

Health Benefits of various spices

Research has found...

Spice	Health Benefits
Allspice	Antiseptic; anesthetic; balances blood sugar
Anise Seed	Alleviates symptoms of asthma and congestion; laxative
Anise Star	Diuretic, reduces gas
Apple Pie Spice	Antibacterial; balances blood sugar; alleviates congestion; sedative
Basil	Anti-inflammatory; antioxidant, strengthens defenses against asthma, osteoarthritis and rheumatoid arthritis
Bay Leaf	Balances blood sugar and retards weight gain; sedative; may help reduce high blood pressure
Cardamom	Reduces heartburn and helps digest grains
Cayenne	Anti-inflammatory; improves circulation; enhances memory; opens respiratory passages
Celery Seed	Helps relieve symptoms of gout, insomnia, and kidney stones
Chili	Anti-inflammatory; improves circulation; enhances memory; opens respiratory passages
Chinese 5 Spice	Improves digestion and promotes intestinal health; anti-inflammatory; antioxidant and antibacterial; stimulates the breakdown of fat cells; relieves congestion, stomach cramps and headaches; balances blood sugar
Chives	May decrease risk of prostate cancer, and reduce cholesterol
Cilantro	Used to regulate digestion and remedy bladder problems; antibacterial that may be an effective natural means of combating salmonella

<u>Cinnamon</u>	Antibacterial; balances blood sugar; alleviates congestion; sedative
<u>Cloves</u>	Painkiller; alleviates diarrhea and nausea
<u>Coriander</u>	Anti-inflammatory; reduces cholesterol; prevents gas; alleviates cramps and gout
<u>Coriander Cumin</u>	Anti-inflammatory; improves circulation; enhances memory; opens respiratory passages; Antibacterial; balances blood sugar; Anti-inflammatory
<u>Cumin</u>	Antiviral; anti-inflammatory; memory enhancer
<u>Dill Weed</u>	Antioxidant; helps prevent growth of bacteria
<u>Fennel</u>	Relieves congestion, stomach cramps and headaches
<u>Fenugreek</u>	Lowers cholesterol; prevents gas; relieves sore throat and congestion; laxative
<u>Garam Masala</u>	Reduces heartburn and helps digest grains; antibacterial; antiviral; anti-inflammatory; balances blood sugar; reduces cholesterol
<u>Garlic</u>	Antibacterial; lowers cholesterol and blood pressure; reduces water retention
<u>Ginger</u>	Antibacterial; improves circulation; stimulates lymph glands; alleviates motion sickness and nausea
<u>Ginger Mustard</u>	Antibacterial; improves circulation; stimulates lymph glands; alleviates motion sickness and nausea; alleviates congestion, bronchitis, sore throat and arthritis; aids digestion of oily and fatty foods
<u>Ginger Spice Blend</u>	Antibacterial; improves circulation; stimulates lymph glands; alleviates motion sickness and nausea
<u>Greek Seasoning</u>	Antibacterial; antioxidant; lowers cholesterol and blood pressure; reduces water retention; alleviates congestion; Improves digestion and promotes intestinal health; anti-inflammatory.

<u>Herbes Provencal</u>	Antioxidant; anti-inflammatory; antimicrobial; nutrient dense; helps digest fatty foods
<u>Italian Seasoning</u>	Antiseptic; reduces high blood pressure; alleviates symptoms of asthma and colds; antibacterial; lowers cholesterol and blood pressure; reduces water retention
<u>Lavender</u>	Used to treat burns, insomnia, anxiety, migraines, symptoms of menopause and to balance blood sugars
<u>Lemon Anise</u>	Alleviates symptoms of asthma and congestion; antiseptic; reduces high blood pressure, antioxidant; promotes kidney and liver health; improves digestion and promotes intestinal health
<u>Lemon Dill Rub</u>	Alleviates symptoms of asthma and congestion; antiseptic; reduces high blood pressure, antioxidant; promotes kidney and liver health; improves digestion and promotes intestinal health
<u>Lemon Grass</u>	promotes digestion of fats, alleviates fevers and menstrual cramps
<u>Lemon Peel</u>	Alleviates congestion; cleaning agent; high in vitamin C
<u>Marjoram</u>	Antibacterial; antioxidant
<u>Mustard</u>	Alleviates congestion, bronchitis, sore throat and arthritis
<u>Onion</u>	Antiseptic, reduces high blood pressure, alleviates symptoms of asthma and colds
<u>Orange Peel</u>	Helps prevent scurvy and colds; high in vitamin C
<u>Oregano</u>	Antibacterial, antioxidant, nutrient rich
<u>Paprika</u>	Helps heal canker sores; improves circulation; alleviates symptoms of colds and kidney infections
<u>Parsley</u>	Antioxidant; helps neutralize certain carcinogens; improves eyesight; promotes kidney and liver health
<u>Peppercorns</u>	Improves digestion and promotes intestinal health; anti-

	inflammatory; antioxidant and antibacterial; stimulates the breakdown of fat cells
Peppermint	Muscle relaxant; digestive aide; antibacterial; antioxidant; anti-inflammatory
Poppy Seed	Stimulates appetite
Poultry Seasoning	Aids digestion of oily and fatty foods; antioxidant, anti-inflammatory, improves brain function
Red Pepper	Anti-inflammatory; improves circulation; enhances memory; opens respiratory passages
Rosemary	Stimulates the immune system; improves circulation; improves digestion
Rosemary Garlic	Stimulates the immune system; improves circulation; improves digestion; antibacterial; lowers cholesterol
Sage	Aids digestion of oily and fatty foods; antioxidant, anti-inflammatory, improves brain function
Sea Salt	Slows bacterial growth; alleviates sore muscles and sore throats
Tarra Cardamom	Anti-fungal; anti-oxidant; sedative; reduces heartburn; helps digest grains
Tarragon	Anti-fungal; anti-oxidant; sedative
Thyme	Anti-oxidant; anti-inflammatory; anti-microbial; nutrient dense; helps digest fatty foods
Turmeric	Anti-oxidant; reduces cholesterol, inflammation, and indigestion

This and more information and research found at:

http://www.smithandtruslow.com/health_benefits.php

Be sure and read the first chapter of Dr. Pray's *I Don't Go With Fat Boys* on the following pages. Order your copy at www.novolife.net or call toll free 866-759-3746

1

Humble Beginnings as a Fat Boy

The year was 1964. I was 11-years-old and in the sixth
grade at Northeast Elementary School in Broken Arrow,
Oklahoma. And I was madly in love with Paula Forbes.

I had always been crazy about girls, ever since I was a
little kid. But Paula was different. She was special. She was
so pretty and so mature for an 11-year-old. Back in those
days, when a boy liked a girl as much as I liked Paula, he
asked her to go steady. So one day while we were out on
the playground at recess, I mustered up all my courage
and asked Paula if she would go steady with me. She said
yes! I gave her some kind of silly little ring (that probably
came from a bubble gum machine), and Paula became my
girlfriend. We were going steady.

I was on top of the world. I lived and breathed Paula. I
dreamed about her during the day in school and at night in
bed. The only time I ever saw her in person was in school
or out on the playground. So when the school year drew to
a close, I became depressed. Don't get me wrong – I loved
summertime and my break from school, but that year, I didn't
want summer to come because I knew I'd never see Paula.

But summer came anyway. In those days, boys didn't call girls on the telephone (at least not in Broken Arrow, Oklahoma). We didn't have cell phones, text messaging, or chat rooms, and the only tweets came from the birds outside. That summer, I literally never spoke to Paula. I thought about her every day.

That was the longest summer of my childhood. Three months crept by, and finally the new school year was just around the corner. I couldn't wait for school to start. I had never been so excited about the beginning of a new school year. I wanted to see Paula again more than anything.

On my first day of seventh grade at Oakcrest School, I didn't see Paula all morning. *What if her family moved away during the summer? What if I never see her again?* I was a nervous wreck. Finally, it was time for recess.

I ran out on the playground, dodging the dodgeball game and leaping over a game of hopscotch. I had no time for games. I was on a mission. I had to find Paula.

Then I saw her on the other side of the playground. She was standing with two other girls, and although her back was to me, I recognized her immediately. I knew that was my Paula. My heart fluttered.

I ran up to Paula with a big, dumb grin on my face and tapped her on the shoulder.

"Paula, Paula, do you want to go steady again this year?" I asked.

She turned around, looked me up and down, and said, "Ew, I don't go with fat boys."

I was crushed. I had never experienced such harsh rejection. I didn't know what to say, so I didn't say anything. I just turned and walked away. For the rest of the day, I wallowed in my misery. I kept my head down on my desk during class. It took all I had to hold back the tears.

When I got home and saw my mom, the levee broke and my pent-up tears burst forth. I told my mom what Paula had said -- that she didn't go with fat boys. Up until that moment, I didn't even realize that I was fat. I guess I had gained some weight over the summer, but I didn't notice. I was a kid. I didn't care if I had a little pudginess around the waistline. I simply never thought about it.

To make matters worse, my brother, who is 18 months older than I am, heard about what happened and gave me a nickname: *Fat Boy*. The nickname stuck for several years and really got under my skin. My brother was a skinny kid, and I was a Fat Boy, unworthy of a girlfriend. Pretty girls don't go with fat boys. I had learned this fact of life the hard way.

My mom, being an insightful mother, noticed how hard I was taking the unexpected break-up. Mom had a weight problem, too. She belonged to the TOPS club in Tulsa. TOPS stands for Taking Off Pounds Sensibly. It's a non-profit weight loss support organization that was founded in 1948.

The TOPS club is still in existence today. In fact, I recently spoke at their state convention. TOPS clubs across the nation educate members about nutrition and exercise. You can join a TOPS club in your area for a low annual fee. The groups meet once a week to provide education, support, encouragement, and incentive to those who want to lose weight.

My mom took me to join the TOPS club in Broken Arrow. I guess she didn't want to take her son along to her own TOPS meetings. I didn't quite understand why then, but I understand now. Like other support group meetings, TOPS club meetings can get pretty personal. People talk about their weight problems as well as the issues behind them. My mom wanted us to have different support groups so that we could speak freely without fear of judging or being judged.

So, at age 12, I started going to TOPS meetings by

myself. We met every Thursday night, and we had a weigh-in before the meeting. When the meeting started, if you lost weight, you called out, "I'm TOPS." If your weight stayed the same, you said, "I'm a turtle." And if you had gained weight during the past week, you had to announce, "I'm a pig." And, everyone said "Oink, oink!" They don't do that at meetings today, thank God times have changed. TOPS is a great organization. I'm thankful my mother introduced me.

The TOPS club taught me about accountability. You learn about accountability quickly when you have to say "I'm a pig" in front of a group of people! Such a practice may sound a bit cruel, but accountability is an important aspect of weight loss. When you have to answer to another person or a group about your eating habits, your exercise, and your weight loss efforts, you learn a lot more about yourself. The back-and-forth dialogue can reveal many epiphanies that you wouldn't experience otherwise.

TOPS also provided incentive to lose weight. My biggest incentive was the cash. Each week, everybody put some money in a pot. Whoever lost the most weight that week would win the cash pot. I won several times.

My mom provided added incentive. Whenever I lost weight, she would make the dinner of my choice. If I wanted to pig out on homemade brownies that night, that was okay – as long as I had lost weight that week. Looking back, that doesn't seem like the healthiest incentive program. But I guess it worked for me as a kid.

My mom and TOPS helped me lose a lot of weight. My first diet was the grapefruit diet. I simply ate a whole grapefruit before each meal. Many times, since I was in an inspired weight loss mode, I'd skip the meal after eating the grapefruit. I lost more weight than any kid in TOPS in the entire state. I lost 24 whole pounds. It may not sound like much, but that was a lot of weight for a 12-year-old!

Later that year, I was crowned the Tiny TOP Prince of Oklahoma. I received a crown, a robe, and an Oklahoma Tiny TOP Prince banner. I got an all-expense paid trip to the international TOPS convention in Toronto. When I walked down the aisle representing my state, hundreds of people cheered for me. It was a great feeling.

Suddenly I felt like a whole new person. I was no longer a Fat Boy. I was slim and confident. I went through several girlfriends. As for Paula – *Paula who?*

Little did I know, this was just the beginning a long stretch of yo-yo dieting and weight loss programs. My weight went up and down over and over again from then on out. I had gotten over Paula, but that fateful day on the playground affected my psyche at a deep level. After that day, I was always worried about being the Fat Boy. Even when I was skinny, I was worried about being fat.

When I started high school, I was extremely concerned about my weight. I was still crazy about girls, and I thought that every girl was thinking about how fat I was. Now, I look back at my high school photos and see that I was not overweight. It was all in my mind – but the mind is a powerful thing.

My confidence, which was sky-high when I was Tiny TOP Prince of Oklahoma, slowly faded as I got older. By the time I finished high school, my self-esteem was very low. I felt like I would be a paranoid Fat Boy for the rest of my life.

I married quickly – when I was 19. The marriage lasted for only a year, and I quickly married again. I was constantly concerned about my weight yet slowly gaining weight. I'd go on a diet, lose a few pounds, and then gain them all back plus a couple more.

Over the years, I tried over 100 diets. I got the same result with each one. I've lost at least 2,300 pounds in my lifetime. With each failed diet, I became a little more discouraged. *Maybe I'm just destined to be a Fat Boy for my entire life,* I'd think.

My second marriage lasted 17 years, and I blame my weight for my second divorce. My second wife was slim like a model – and beautiful like a model, too. When we divorced, she made a list of all the reasons why she wanted a divorce, including all of my faults. Guess what was on that list?

- *You're FAT!*

I felt the pain of Paula Forbes' playground proclamation all over again. This time around, I was truly heart-broken. I had lost my beautiful wife, my life partner of 17 years – not some girl on the playground who I only saw a few minutes a day during the school year. And my wife's ring didn't come from a bubble gum machine!

I lost a lot of weight after my second divorce. The irony is that I wasn't even very fat at the time. Sure, I was a little overweight, but at 6'1" and 230 pounds, I wasn't obese. But my wife thought I was fat, and she let me know. In my mind, I became Fat Boy all over again.

I stayed thin for a few years, but when the weight started to come back, as it always did, I lost all hope. I was the Fat Boy, and there was nothing I could do about it. What was the use in trying? I quickly ballooned up to 287 pounds. My waist got up to 48 inches. I was getting ready to buy my first 50-inch pair of pants when I decided, "I'm not going to do this!"

I should also mention that I was actually teaching nutrition at my local college when I gained all this weight. There I was standing in front of a classroom at nearly 300 pounds, lecturing about weight loss. Can you imagine how guilty I felt?

I had to do something. I was tired of feeling guilty, and I refused to buy 50-inch pants. I decided to try a new diet called the Atkins diet. I lost quite a bit of weight on this low-carb, high-protein diet. In fact, I was so impressed by the diet that I started teaching classes about it. I was a true Atkins aficionado.

Then a funny thing happened: My 17-year-old daughter introduced me to a whole new way of looking at nutrition. At the time, she was having some health problems, primarily due to hormone imbalances. She was also hypoglycemic. She'd have "weak attacks" when her blood sugar got too low. As the Atkins aficionado, I thought, "No problem! I'll fix her right up with my low-carb diet."

My daughter had other plans. She did her own research and discovered the book *Fasting and Eating for Health: A Medical Doctor's Program for Conquering Disease* by Joel Fuhrman, MD. After reading the book, my daughter informed me that she was going on a 21-day water fast, consuming absolutely nothing but water for three whole weeks.

"Are you crazy?" I asked her.

My daughter was undeterred, so I agreed to read Dr. Fuhrman's book. And, you know what, it all made sense to me. Sure, I was still skeptical, and some of Dr. Fuhrman's claims seemed a bit outlandish. For example, Dr. Fuhrman writes:

Therapeutic fasting accelerates the healing process and allows the body to recover from serious disease in a dramatically short period of time. In my practice I have seen fasting eliminate lupus and arthritis, remove chronic skin conditions such as psoriasis and eczema, heal the digestive tract in patients with ulcerative colitis and Crohn's disease, and quickly eliminate cardiovascular diseases such as high blood pressure and angina. In these cases the recoveries were permanent: fasting enabled longtime disease sufferers to unchain themselves from their multiple toxic drugs and even eliminate the need for surgery, which was recommended to some of them as their only solution.

Despite my lingering doubts, I supported my daughter's decision. She was determined to go through with the fast, and I was determined to make sure she didn't damage her body in the process. We had blood work done before she started the fast, and I monitored her numbers throughout the entire three-week period.

During the fast, I checked on her constantly, which turned out to be an easy task. She basically lounged around and did nothing for three weeks. She didn't have the energy or strength to do anything. Near the end of the fast, she couldn't even read because her ability to focus had disappeared.

But she made it three weeks without consuming anything but water – and she lost a lot of weight. Additionally, the fast normalized her hormones and blood sugar level. She followed the advice in Dr. Fuhrman's book, and she healed herself. I was impressed – very impressed.

It wasn't long before my daughter bought a copy of Dr. Fuhrman's book *Eat to Live: The Revolutionary Formula for Fast and Sustained Weight Loss.*

"I'm going to start on this diet now, dad," she said, showing me the book.

She told me about the basics of Dr. Fuhrman's whole food diet.

"That won't work," I said smugly. "It's not a high-protein diet. In fact, it's almost all carbs. That won't work at all."

"Well, I'm going to do it, dad," she said. And I knew she would.

I was still teaching the Atkins diet, and my own daughter was going against my own advice. I was insulted! To make matters worse, since I wasn't exactly supporting my daughter, my new wife decided to go on the diet with her. Then I was even more insulted.

They went out and bought a bunch of nuts, seeds, fruits, vegetables, and beans. That night they made dinner and brought a plate into my office.

"Why are we eating this?" I protested. "It's all carbs! I can't believe you two are doing this!"

"Dad, just read the book," my daughter pleaded.

So I grabbed the book with the intention of picking

it apart, critiquing it, and telling my wife and daughter everything that was wrong with it. With red ink pen in one hand and a fine-tooth comb in the other, I started reading.

I soon noticed that Dr. Fuhrman backed up all of his statements with research. I was so intent on proving him wrong that I looked up every single study he cited in *Eat to Live.* The harder I worked to prove him wrong, the more I agreed with his ideas. By the time I finished reading the book, I said, "You know what, this guy has it all figured out."

At that point, I had no choice: I had to try Dr. Fuhrman's whole food diet. I stopped counting carbs and started eating large salads. The results were amazing. I immediately dropped extra pounds and went down to near my ideal weight.

Then I made a big mistake: I went to a TOPS club meeting and told them that I would never be fat again. I told the members about Dr. Fuhrman's whole food diet. I told them that I had learned how to eat for the first time – that the whole food diet was God's diet plan for us all, the way we were designed to eat. Armed with this knowledge, I told them that I'd never be fat again.

Nine months later, I was fat again. The whole food diet worked for a while. Then Christmas came around. Since I was at my ideal weight, I decided that it was okay for me to have extra turkey and dressing. Then I reasoned that it was okay to have a piece of mom's homemade banana pie.

Mmm, that's good pie. One more piece can't hurt. After all, it's Christmas!

I gained a pound or two that week and a pound or two the next week. Over the next 90 days, I gained 30 pounds.

Looking in the mirror, I wondered how this could've happened. At the TOPS meeting, I said that I'd never be fat again. I had finally learned how to eat. Dr. Fuhrman's book gave me the perfect diet plan – and I still blew it. What happened?

That's when I realized that I was addicted to junk food – processed foods, refined foods, whatever you want to call them – high-calorie foods with low nutritional value. I started studying addiction and alcoholism, and I recognized the addictive patterns in my own life. I wasn't addicted to drugs or alcohol, but I certainly had a problem with high-fat, high-sugar food. I'm just as addicted to refined food as an alcoholic is addicted to booze.

I had to find a way to break the cycle of addiction. It's not just about knowing how to eat. If it were that simple, we'd all avoid junk food and not have any weight problems. The alcoholics who realize that alcohol is the source of their problems would simply quit drinking. But it's not that easy. We have to find some way to break the cycle of addiction.

At this point, I went back to Dr. Fuhrman's first book, *Fasting and Eating for Health*. I remembered how my daughter's fast had normalized her body's natural functions. It was almost as if the fast had rebooted her system. I wondered if a fast would help me to break my food addiction.

I learned everything that I could about fasting, cleansing, and detoxifying the body. I knew that I couldn't go on a three-week water fast. I had a business to run. I had patients to see and classes to teach. I had responsibilities that required my attention and energy. A shorter cleanse, however, would be feasible.

Working with a partner, Dr. Jeff Cartwright, I developed a healthy seven-day cleanse that allowed me to reap the benefits of a fast while maintaining my energy level. The program includes a cleansing formula to release toxins from nervous tissue and fat tissue; a metabolic boosting formula to enhance the body's ability to burn fat; and a meal replacement formula to maintain energy levels.

When I did my first cleanse a couple of years ago, I lost 13 pounds in seven days! My blood pressure dropped, my triglycerides dropped, my cholesterol dropped, and my blood sugar dropped. Best of all, I was able to break my addiction to junk food.

My cravings for burgers, fries, and cola disappeared. Before the cleanse, there was no way you could get me to eat a big bowl of fresh fruit or green vegetables because I was so addicted to junk food. That's all I craved and all I wanted to eat. After the cleanse, I didn't crave junk food anymore. I actually craved the steamed broccoli and other healthy foods.

Once I gave my body a chance to reboot itself, so to speak, my cravings changed; my body started to crave truly healthy food. My sense of taste changed, and the flavors of foods seemed to change. It was incredible! For the first time I could remember, eating healthy was actually easy and even enjoyable.

The modern American diet consists of refined foods that are full of toxins. Meats and dairy products contain pharmaceuticals, pesticides, and hormones. Processed foods contain all sorts of synthetic chemicals with names you can't pronounce. Even fresh fruits and vegetables are contaminated with toxins. And now we have to worry about genetically engineered foods that are introducing brand new inflammatory proteins into our bodies.

We're also exposed to toxins in the water we drink and the air we breathe. It's impossible to avoid toxins. The body does its best to process and eliminate toxins, but it can only handle so much. When you're taking in toxins faster than your body can process them, your body must store them in fat tissue. Your body fat is actually saving your life by holding onto to all those dangerous toxins!

Exposure to a high level of toxins – like the toxins in the typical American diet – overtaxes the body's natural defense system. The body is working so hard to process and store toxins that you don't have any energy left for important activities like exercise. However, when you detoxify and reduce your toxic load, your body can let go of the excess fat. There's no need for it any longer. After a cleanse, your fat will melt away, you'll have more energy, and you'll feel great.

After my first cleanse, I knew I was onto something big. I had broken my junk food addiction. But I also knew that, inevitably, the addiction would return as it always had. Addiction is cunning, baffling, and powerful. I had to develop a plan to keep the addiction at bay.

My plan revolves around accountability, mindfulness, careful monitoring of my weight, and quick action when the addiction begins to resurface.

Nobody's perfect. I'm certainly not perfect, and statistics show that I'm like most people. Over 98 percent of diets fail. Each year, Americans spend $60 billion on weight loss programs that have a two percent success rate.

Most people cannot follow a diet plan for long. A holiday rolls around, or they go out to eat, and they slip up. After gaining a few pounds, they become discouraged and eventually give up. I went through this cycle of yo-yo dieting for nearly 40 years before I realized how to make it work.

I monitor my weight carefully, and when I mess up – when I gain a couple of pounds – I go on a mini-cleanse to nip the addiction in the bud. Instead of becoming discouraged, I lose the weight that I regained while keeping my body healthy.

I monitor my patients' weight carefully, too. My patients weigh-in each week. When patients gain a couple of pounds, I ask them what happened. If they went to a wedding over the weekend, perhaps they overate and gained an extra pound. I hold them accountable and encourage them to realize where they went wrong.

Then I tell them, "That's okay. I've done the same thing myself many times." Nobody's perfect. I offer them a solution: a mini-cleanse and a couple of days of strict adherence to the whole food diet. By the end of the week, they've lost the pound that they gained plus another. This system works, even for those of us who are not perfect.

Like many of you, I love to eat. It's my favorite thing to do. I love junk food, and I still eat it when I can. But I know how easily I become addicted to it again -- and if that happens, then my cholesterol goes up, my triglycerides go up, my blood sugar goes up, my blood pressure goes up, I get fat, I get lazy, and I become discouraged. Suddenly, I'm addicted to junk food once again. I can't allow that to happen.

At the same time, I know that I will mess up, and that's okay. I try to stick to my whole food diet 90 percent of the time; 10 percent of the time, I allow myself to slip and eat junk food. I call it the 10 percent plan. Whenever I gain weight, a mini-cleanse resets my body chemistry before addiction can take hold. Then I go back to the whole food diet.

Instead of falling off the wagon, becoming discouraged, and reentering the cycle of addiction, my patients and I are able to continue moving forward without feeling guilty when we mess up. We never totally fall off the wagon.

Not everyone agrees with my weight loss plan. Some nutritionists feel that I'm allowing my patients to mess up. But guess what -- people are going to mess up 98 percent of the time anyway. At least I have an answer and plan of action for them when they do. It's not a perfect weight loss plan, but it works for imperfect people like me.

This plan has provided the solution to my own weight loss problems, and it has worked for many others as well. My patients have a 70 percent success rate for weight loss.

Most diets fail because people eventually get hungry and overeat or splurge on junk food. Here's the most important part of my weight loss plan: Never allow yourself to get hungry. Eat until you are stuffed. It's not how much you eat but what you eat that matters. That's where the whole food diet comes in.

Kale	1000	Tofu	86	Bananas	30
Collards	1000	Sweet Potatoes	83	Chicken Breast	27
Bok Choy	824	Apples	76	Eggs	27
Spinach	739	Peaches	73	Low Fat Yogurt, plain	26
Cabbage	481	Kidney Beans	71	Corn	25
Red Pepper	420	Green Peas	70	Almonds	25
Romaine Lettuce	389	Lentils	68	Whole Wheat Bread	25
Broccoli	342	Pineapple	64	Feta Cheese	21
Cauliflower	295	Avocado	64	Whole Milk	20
Green Peppers	258	Oatmeal	53	Ground Beef	20
Artichoke	244	Mangoes	51	White Pasta	18
Carrots	240	Cucumbers	50	White Bread	18
Asparagus	234	Soybeans	48	Peanut Butter	18
Strawberries	212	Sunflower Seeds	45	Apple Juice	16
Tomatoes	164	Brown Rice	41	Swiss Cheese	15
Plums	157	Salmon	39	Potato Chips	11
Blueberries	130	Shrimp	38	American Cheese	10
Iceberg Lettuce	110	Skim Milk	36	Vanilla Ice Cream	9
Orange	109	White Potatoes	31	French Fries	7
Cantaloupe	100	Grapes	31	Olive Oil	2
Flax Seeds	44	Walnuts	29	Cola	1

Dr. Fuhrman has ranked foods according to their nutrient density. Nutrient density is the ratio of nutrients to calories. In ranking various foods, Dr. Fuhrman considers all the vitamins, nutrients, and phytonutrients (plant nutrients) in 1000 calories of the given food, then he assigns a nutrient density ranking of 1 to 1000. Here's a sample of Dr. Fuhrman's nutrient density scores from his website, drfuhrman.com: *(See Table above)*

If you want to lose weight, you simply eat more nutrient-dense foods and avoid the foods with lower nutrient-density scores. It's that simple. Forget counting calories or carbs. Eat foods with a high ratio of nutrients to calories. You'll not only lose weight, but you'll also gain health.

Nutrient-dense whole foods contain proteins, fats, carbs,

water, fiber, vitamins, minerals, and phytonutrients. Dark green, leafy vegetables like kale, collards, and spinach are the most nutrient-dense foods. Pop-eye had it right! You cannot eat too much spinach. In fact, the more spinach you eat, the more weight you'll lose. Each bite makes you healthier. You should try to eat a pound of raw leafy greens each day. You'll see amazing results.

A full pound of spinach contains only 100 calories. You could eat 10 pounds of spinach every day and still lose weight (although I've never heard of anyone eating 10 pounds of spinach in a single day). That's the beauty of this plan: You never go hungry. You fill up on healthy foods and never allow yourself to get hungry.

Now, let's compare a pound of spinach to a pound of olive oil: One pound of olive oil has 2300 calories, and all of those calories come from 100% fat. Olive oil also contains some vitamins, but not in a quantity significant enough to raise its nutrient density score.

In recent years, olive oil has become popular among many dieters because of the Mediterranean diet. However, the Mediterranean diet works because of its focus on fruits, vegetables, and whole grains – not because of olive oil. Of course, olive oil, as a monosaturated fat, is healthier than saturated fats and polysaturated fats, but the fact remains that it's still extracted fat. If you're trying to lose weight, you should avoid excess oils and fats. We'll discuss the different types of fat in more detail in chapter 6.

When you study the nutrient density of foods, it soon becomes clear that God had a natural plan for us to remain healthy and thin naturally. The most nutrient-dense foods are also the lowest calorie foods. On the other hand, the most popular foods in the modern American diet are high in calories but low in nutrients. These foods are not natural. They have been refined, processed, and stripped of their nutritional value.

When you constantly eat foods devoid of nutritional value, your body craves more food to fill that void. That's why it's so easy to overeat and consume far too many calories when you're eating refined foods.

Most diets fail because the dieter's will power fails. Will power fails because people get hungry. My solution is simple: Don't let yourself get hungry! Eat, and eat until you're stuffed – but make sure that you're filling up on nutrient-dense foods.

My patients often call me in a panic after weeks of doing well in my weight loss program. "Help!" they say. "We're going out to eat at the steak house. What am I supposed to do?"

I tell them to plan ahead. Eat an apple before you go out to eat. The skin of an apple contains a natural appetite suppressant. It will help fill you up before you order at the restaurant, and you'll eat half as much.

When you order, start with a salad. Sometimes I even eat two salads when I go out to eat. I ask my server to leave off the croutons and add extra tomatoes, and I never choose a high-fat salad dressing. I usually order a low-fat balsamic dressing on the side. A healthy salad becomes unhealthy when you drown it in a high-fat dressing. Try to fill up on salad, and you won't want that slice of apple pie for dessert.

You can make healthy choices even when you're eating out in a restaurant. In a steak house, for instance, you can order the shrimp kabobs and a plain baked potato. After eating the apple, the salad, and the shrimp kabobs, you should feel satisfied. If you're still hungry, order another side of vegetables. Just don't allow yourself to get hungry.

Most popular diets work on the principle of calorie restriction, and dieters will eventually get hungry, overeat, and give up. A calorie restriction diet will help you lose weight if you stick to it, but how long will you stick to it?

Forget counting calories. Remember, what you're eating is more important than how much you're eating. Granted, you could lose weight on a pizza diet, a pasta diet, or even a chocolate diet if you restricted your calories.

If you're burning more calories than you consume, you'll lose weight. It's simple math. Here's the generic formula for weight loss based on calorie restriction: Multiply your current body weight times 10. If you weigh 200 pounds, the number would be 2,000; that's how many daily calories it takes to maintain your current weight. If you want to lose weight, cut your daily calorie intake by 400. By the end of the week, you will have lost a pound.

You can eat pizza three times a day, and if you're consuming 1,600 hundred calories or less with a current weight of 200 pounds, you'll still lose a pound a week. But the problem is that you'll eventually get hungry and eat more pizza. Your body will crave nutrients, and you'll overeat. With my plan, you don't have to count calories – and you don't have to go hungry.

In most cases, calorie-restriction diets actually promote weight gain. When people are on the diet, their metabolic rate slows down because they're eating less. When they go off the diet, their slower metabolism causes them to get even heavier than they were before they started the diet.

The Atkins diet revolves around counting carbs rather than calories. Carbs are severely restricted in the Atkins diet. Can you lose weight on the Atkins diet? Sure, but as soon as you go off the diet, you'll gain the weight back. In addition, the Atkins diet is not healthy. You're missing out on plant-based nutrients and health benefits.

The high-protein Atkins diet encourages consumption of meat products, and as you will learn from this book, a diet based on meat products has serious consequences for your health. Plant-based diets are much healthier. Plants not only provide the three energy producing macronutrients (protein, fat, and carbohydrates) as well as, vitamins, minerals, and water, but they also provide the essential micronutrients –phytonutrients.

Researchers are just now beginning to understand the importance of phytonutrients – natural chemicals that you can get only from consuming whole plant foods. Phytonutrients in fruits and vegetables act as powerful antioxidants; they neutralize free radicals in your body that cause oxidative damage and promote inflammation and aging. A plant-based diet will provide your body with everything you need to be healthy and prevent cancer, heart disease, diabetes, fibromyalgia, and other chronic diseases.

In searching for the perfect weight loss plan, I stumbled upon the perfect plan for holistic health. If you follow the advice in this book, you will not only lose weight but also reduce your risk of disease, extend your lifespan, and enjoy your new lease on life with more energy and vitality.

You will learn how to move right, eat right, and think right. If your head's not in the right place, then your weight loss is doomed from the beginning. A positive attitude is crucial. Successful weight loss is one-third diet, one-third exercise, and one-third mentality.

I understand your frustration. I feel your pain. I've been there myself. I will show you how to maintain a positive attitude even after you gain a couple of pounds. You don't have to fall back into the cycle of addiction. With a solid plan, you will overcome your addiction to junk food for good.

Like I said, not everyone agrees with my weight loss plan. Not everyone understands my weight loss plan. They don't understand what it's like to lose weight, gain it all back, go on another diet, lose weight, and gain it all back again. They're in that fortunate 2 percent of people who can stick to a healthy diet all the time. I'm in that 98 percent that will fail time after time, and that's why I developed this weight loss plan for imperfect people.

When I went on my first diet at age 12, I never imagined that I'd make a career out of weight loss. Now, weight loss is not just my career; it's my life's mission. Obesity is the biggest health threat in the United States. Approximately eight out of ten Americans are overweight, and nearly forty percent are approaching morbidly obese. That means your weight is literally killing you!

As a weight loss specialist, I have to practice what I preach. I have overcome my addiction to refined foods, and I'm enjoying eating healthy, whole foods every day. My weight is down to 210 and slowly dropping even lower. With each bite of spinach, I become a little healthier.

I still love to eat, and I'll be the first to admit it: I still go out to eat and sample the junk food occasionally. But now I have a solid plan for when I mess up – and that plan is working so well for me that I want to share it with you.

It's time for a new beginning and a new life. Are you ready?

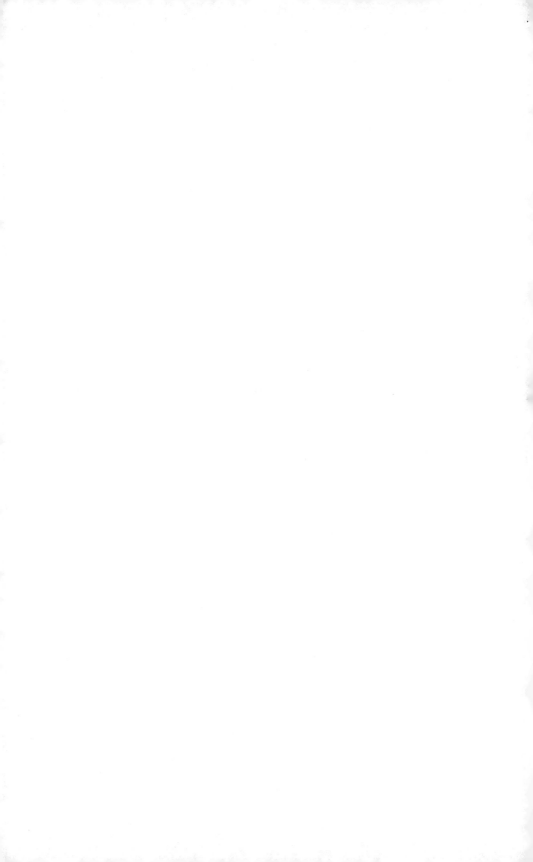

CPSIA information can be obtained at www.ICGtesting.com
Printed in the USA
LVOW090304141111

254830LV00002B/9/P